Clear You:

Acne Healing Solution

Stephen J. Rodriguez, HHC

Clear You: Acne Healing Solution

Printed in the United States of America.

ISBN: 1500768839
ISBN-13: 978-1500768836

DEDICATION

To the women in my life and the God
that I adore. Without you, this is all meaningless.

ACKNOWLEDGMENTS

With the emotional toll that acne takes on individuals every minute of every day I felt it was time to do something about it. For everyone out there that has suffered, will suffer, or is suffering from acne. I want to thank you for your endurance and perseverance through such an emotionally debilitating condition. You are truly my heroes. I would also like to thank Joshua Rosenthal and everyone at the Institute for Integrative Nutrition. Your work is far from complete and the effect of what you do will truly ripple through time. Thank you.

CONTENTS

Acknowledgments

Start Here

Part One: The Story On Acne

Part Two: Acne Misinformation

Part Three: But I Like Cookies

Part Four: Acne Eradication

Part Five: Life Beyond Acne

Part Six: Additional Aids & Info

About the Author

START HERE

Welcome to the *CLEAR YOU: Acne Healing Solution* book! I'm your host Stephen Rodriguez and I'd like to personally thank you for your interest in yourself and your face. Chances are you wouldn't have picked this book up if you weren't interested in getting rid of your acne.

If you're like most people, acne isn't something you may understand very well. To be honest, acne isn't really understood by anyone. Sure there are plenty of old wives tales about not eating this and making sure to eat that, but there is a lot more confusion than hard facts.

Does ice make acne smaller? Does it make it worse? What about the old toothpaste remedy, surely this is the cure all of all things acne. Ever tried rubbing cayenne pepper on your pimple? These things can't be the best solutions. Surely in an age of modern science where we've learned to master the atom and gone to the moon just to never go back, you'd think that we'd have an answer to the question of acne.

Not even the best and brightest in the medical community understand acne very well. For a disease that's been around a few thousand years, you'd think we would know more about what to do about it; but, alas most are clueless. The goal of this book is to shed some light on acne in a light hearted, fun way, and hopefully provide some answers to the question of how to reduce or even eliminate it.

If you've ever been marginalized in a doctor's office, treated like a number, or been dismissed as paranoid because of acne, then this book is what you've been looking for. Other books that have talked about getting control of acne tend to lean heavily on the supplement and product side of things. Authors will be paid to write about a product or supplement that may or may not help you. It's a gross conflict of interest for an author, or anyone for that matter, to sing the praises of a product that he or she is not willing to use themselves and are only paid to endorse.

I'm not here to sell my one of a kind supplement, or my secret topical agent derived from the root of a banana tree and some sacred mushroom from a mountain top in Tibet.

I'm here to provide simple, easy to use ideas that anyone can use to get acne whooped in a shorter period of time, and keep it off. It is my sole purpose to get you on your way to complete acne reduction and elimination. You can take control of your body and enjoy the *clear you* you've always been capable of being.

Here's how to use the book. This book can be read front to back or it can be read in different sections. The table of contents lays out individual subjects in six different parts that may or may not be relevant to your specific situation. If something works for you, wonderful! If it doesn't, no worries. You will find something that will give you some if not a full measure of relief.

One person's food is another person's poison. There is no one size fits all approach here. One size fits all approaches don't work. If you've ever seen a pair of yoga pants on the rack, you'll quickly understand that it is impossible for a one size fits all approach to work with anything. There is no way everyone will fit in those pants. That's actually ok. You know why? It has everything to do with the unique individual you are. You are a person with unique life experiences, unique fingerprints, and a unique perspective.

Your body is unique. You may share ancestry with a particular people group, or you may be a mix of several races. Regardless, it doesn't matter if you belong to a particular group or have mixed heritage. Your individuality is simply that—your own. Your body won't behave or react like that of the next person. It's the reason why husbands and wives don't always enjoy the same kinds of foods, or why they can look at the same situation and interpret it several different ways. It's the reason why even among siblings, with the same set of parents, both individual people won't see things eye to eye all the time. It's impossible for them to do so. Nature never intended for two individuals to be alike. We were intended to celebrate our uniqueness, one person at a time.

Throughout the chapters you'll see segments called *My Acne Horror Story*. You can read them while you're reading the chapter, read them by themselves all at once, or any other way you so desire. You can even ignore them if you want. It's all up to you. Everyone whose story I wrote down, all dealt with acne at the most inopportune times. For some of them it hit before their wedding. For others, it was just something they always had and couldn't do anything about.

In them you'll get a chance to see how someone else has suffered from acne just like you. Some of these stories are light hearted and others are really embarrassing. All of them represent the varied experiences that people have had with acne. Everyone in the stories are real people. They were all interviewed in person and were all willing to share their stories. Only their first names are used so they won't have to suffer any more indignity at the hands of acne.

Unfortunately, this book wasn't written when these people had their acne experiences, so their stories aren't testimonials, but they do give some perspective and may help you see some patterns related to what we're talking about in the text. So there you have it. Welcome to the book and you're on your way to a new *CLEAR YOU!*

Part One:

The Story on Acne

1:
A QUICK SUMMARY

Acne. That one word strikes fear into the hearts of teenagers, adults, and soon to be brides everywhere. Those glowing pus filled orbs of swollen glory are not something to be trifled with. It seems like if you just look at a zit, it'll explode. Acne is one of those things in life that seems completely avoidable for some people, and completely inevitable for others.

Has anyone ever asked the question, "Why?" Why does acne seem to strike randomly? Why do you always seem to get a zit right before some major life event? (Brides can relate). Why is it that acne only occurs mainly in the developed world and not developing nations? Does anyone have answers to these questions?

What about acne medication? It seems to work for a little while and then it just stops. That's when acne comes back with a vengeance regardless of the kind of medication you're taking. If you're someone that has tried and tried again to get rid of your acne, these questions have probably crossed your mind at some point in time. Okay, maybe not the question about acne in the developing world, but definitely the others.

What if there was a way to get rid of your acne without having to use any kind of product? I'm serious. No three step process or facial acid baths required. That means no pills, no supplements, no creams, no soaps, and no super, secret sauce that you can only buy from me. Would you be interested? Your body is already pre-packaged to reverse if not eliminate your acne and I can show you how to do it.

This book is written to do just that. It's written to show you, the person reading this, that you can reduce if not eliminate your acne in days. If you'll take the advice and follow some simple concepts your acne will, at the very least, be reduced in a gentle non-traumatic way. For a lot of you that read this book, you'll take complete control of your acne and never have it be an issue again. Is that a bold statement? Yes it is. However, the last 50 years of research in the area of acne reduction/elimination backs that claim. You can find some of the research footnoted and in the **References and Resources** portion of the book.

Acne is one of those things in life that's like the unwanted house guest that eats all of your food. No matter how polite or mean you are, they just won't leave you alone. You're like, "Come on dude! Go away!" It's really embarrassing when this unwanted house guest happens to show up or stick around whenever you have real guests coming over. Think about it. There he is just sitting on the sofa, taking up all of your couch space with a giant bowl of chips on his beer belly mumbling "hi" between fistfuls of thinly sliced potato.

Can you imagine what someone would think if they saw this happening in your house?

They'd probably be wondering why you haven't done something about this guy. They don't realize that no matter what you've tried, whether it was calling the cops, poisoning him (please don't really do this), or literally throwing him out; he just won't leave!

That's what acne feels like for a lot of people. It's that obnoxious, annoying thing that will not leave you alone no matter what you do. Medicine, therapy, and everything else in between only work for a little while and then stop working for a lot of people. Never mind the emotional shame, or the confidence-killing stares that come from people looking at your acne. This is not something easy to deal with by any means. If someone hasn't struggled with it, they really won't be able to relate.

Imagine going into a job interview at 30 years old and you still have giant zits on your face. You can't tell me that doesn't do anything to your confidence. Of course it does. It's a pain when the person that you're hoping will become your boss decides sub-consciously not to hire you because you're still "a kid". Never mind the fact that you are more than qualified for the position and you've got mad job skills. Nope.

The acne did it. Don't think it happens? It happens all of the time.

Something similar happened to me. The only difference is I got the job. Unfortunately, I also got the comments. When I used to sell life insurance, the gentleman that was over me was in his 60's. One time I had dry skin on my face that was irritating me so like any other normal human being, I tried to get it off my face.

"Don't pick at them, that's how you get more," he said. It would have been more or less ok if it was just he and I in the car. The problem was he made this comment with two other people from the company that were also riding with us. I was so embarrassed. What could I say to him though? Nothing. That was a very demoralizing feeling. Emotionally I got over it a long time ago, but it does go to show how people do notice at times you don't want them to.

As much as people try to ignore the superficial, they just can't. People are constantly making judgments based on looks. Think of a car that has a rusted bumper or fender. Does it run well? Is it reliable? I guarantee that if you take one look at the rust on that bumper, you'll probably make a snap judgment about the engine without even test driving it.

You won't even think that the rust might be just superficial. The engine could be in perfect working order; but, because of a little rust, surely this must be an indicator of more problems with the car. Perhaps even a gremlin will be lurking in the glove compartment. Ever heard the old saying, "Don't judge a book by its cover?" We're constantly making judgments based on first impressions.

If you've got a homeless guy on the side of the road he must have been a lazy bum that didn't work hard so that's the reason why he's homeless, right? Maybe, maybe not. It could be that his house burned down two weeks ago and he hasn't been able to collect his insurance money, or maybe he's a disabled vet that can't find work. There's just no way to tell.

Getting control of your acne requires you to think beyond the surface of your skin. It requires you to go deeper. Acne is not something that happens at the surface. In reality it happens far deeper inside of you in the very depths of your body. We'll get into that later, but before we do...

STEPHEN J. RODRIGUEZ

2:
AN ACNE STORY

Having mini Mt. Everests on your face is not only embarrassing, but socially debilitating. I suffered with acne for over 13 years and used to have huge cystic pimples that were the size of the iris in my eye. It was so aggravating to have blood drip down on my clothing after a zit would rupture and not realize it until I looked in a mirror. I don't mean to be gross, but that's what was happening. Acne isn't pretty. It's ugly! It's so personal! You literally wear this one disease on your face and everyone, I mean everyone can see it for what it is. There's no hiding it.

Makeup may hide discolored skin, but all the makeup in the world can't hide the cysts, nodules, or lumps underneath it.

For me acne, a.k.a. Acne Vulgaris, started when I was about 12 years old and quickly exploded all over my body. I carried it straight into adulthood. I was married with acne. Try having your new bride constantly poking at your face, arms, and back with a needle and a knife. Every place she could find a pimple was fair game. Nothing was off limits. It was torture! Okay, so she really didn't use a knife, it was actually a bobby pin, but it was no less painful. I would beg her to go easy on the poking and the squeezing. She wouldn't. It would hurt so much!

Anyway, as a teenager, I was eventually put on several different kinds of medications including two kinds of pills, one cream, and a liquid that I would massage into my face. We lived close to the Mexican border so my family and I would go into Mexico (back in the days when it was safe) to grab tacos and medication. Acne meds in the U.S. were too expensive even with insurance so it was kind of convenient. In Mexico, you didn't even need a prescription.

Just five bucks and the name of the medication is all it took.

My frustration mounted when after a short time the medicines stopped working as well as they used to. So like everyone else I knew, I tried a ton of different products until my mom settled on Proactiv; that wonderful three step topical system that everyone was ranting and raving about. Guess what happened after I tried it? It worked...only for about a month and then I was back into acne land. I kept using Proactiv even though it stopped working for me and continued with my oral medication. There still wasn't much improvement. Don't get me wrong my acne was almost always reduced at first with each new treatment, but it always came back. It would never completely go away. It was the same cycle every time. I would try a new topical cream, medication, or system, and it would always go from bad acne to clear face back to bad acne. It seemed like an endless roller coaster.

Eventually, my mom decided that I should go see a dermatologist because surely they would have the answers. Never mind the fact that my brother, who also had bad acne, had gone to a dermatologist and saw no reduction in his acne afterward. As a matter of fact, they poked the pimples on his face with a needle at his first visit. He looked like a pro boxer three days after a fight with all sorts of clots and bandaids on his face. Nope, these guys knew what was up. In the dermatologist's office I sat there in the waiting room with the slightest hope that perhaps this man or woman would be the God sent angel from heaven that would provide me with the relief I so desperately needed.

Instead, I got a bug-eyed dude with glasses sitting on his nose who had a mustache and wore a lamp on his head. Rudely he refused to shake my hand after I held it out, and I began to think he was germaphobic. This was already not going well. I was just waiting for the sharp objects to come out, but I soon realized that if he wasn't going to shake my hand, then he probably wasn't going to poke my face. Oh yeah, this was going great. Don't get me wrong, I didn't want my face poked, but if a poked face meant relief, then I was willing to endure it.

"Hello" he said, in a very nasal voice. "How can I help you?" My mom proceeded to tell him about how we were trying blah, blah, blah products, and how they weren't doing a thing for me. The whole explanation took about a minute and a half. It was pretty self-explanatory. Every time I tried medication, it would work then stop.

From that point forward during the visit all he did was eyeball me. Forehead to neck, ear to ear, he did nothing more than talk in his voice recorder in some foreign doctors language that I had no hope of understanding. He looked at my mom, said goodbye, and gave her a prescription. That was it. No questions asked, and no real interaction with me--the victim. No emotional support for the shame. No relating to the patient. It was a very isolating experience.

The entire visit lasted about five minutes and cost my hard working mom $150.00 with her copay, not including the expensive new meds. Mexico anyone? Boy I was on my way now! I'm being sarcastic obviously. That was the first time I felt marginalized by a doctor. I remember feeling so disappointed that my angel of mercy was nothing more than a dude with a light on his head that didn't care whether or not I got better. His goal wasn't to give me control of my acne, though I believe he believed he was helping. At least I hope he was. His main goal with the visit was simply to manage my disease by pumping me full of more and more meds. There had to be another way! As I sat on that thought for a while, life would pass me by and take its course with braces and my high school Homecoming. Got to love orthodontia. Metal mouth here I come! As if I wasn't awkward enough with my pimply skin. That's when something really interesting happened.

My orthodontist told my mom that we had to remove my wisdom teeth otherwise my braces would be a pointless waste of money. This was a procedure I was not looking forward to. I had never been under general anesthesia before and I hated the idea of it. Long story short, the surgeon pulled out my wisdom teeth and I was in a world of pain for the first three days. I couldn't open my mouth very wide and I didn't want to risk opening my stitches. Because of this, I wasn't able to eat anything but foods like soft, steamed vegetables and soups. Guess what happened?

My acne completely cleared up in four days! I'm not talking slight redness here and there mixed with a small pimple. I'm talking pimples,

CLEAR YOU: ACNE HEALING SOLUTION

oil, and redness, all gone! I was floored! My mom, my friends, even my dad who usually keeps to himself commented that my face looked great. "That's kind of weird." I thought to myself. For the first time in a long time I looked good. I felt more confident, which is a big deal for an insecure teenager. That one event left a wrinkle in my brain that I couldn't stop thinking about. Eventually I would suppress the memory of that experience, but I couldn't ignore what had happened.

I started to ask people that I knew in the medical community whether or not diet and acne were related. As if in one chorus and song, they all gave a resounding...No. Some would say maybe, but that it was likely there was no connection. If that was the case, then why did my acne clear up in four days of not eating what I normally ate? Once again I brushed off the experience and went on with my life.

When I was 17, my sister in law to be introduced me to an aesthetician (Aus-Te-Tishon). Basically, this person's job is to rehabilitate your skin by utilizing different treatments that include using lasers, creams, scalpels, and acids. Let's not forget the little poker. That's probably not the name of it, but that's what I called it. The scalpels were my favorite part.

Here's how the visit would go. First, she would steam my face with water vapor. According to her, this was to open the pores on my face, but I like to think that she was tenderizing me before cutting. After being tenderized for 10 minutes, she would pull out the scalpel and cut open every zit. It made the sound of tearing paper when she would open me up. It's weird that you get used to someone cutting in to you with a medical device that's used for major surgery. It's like they're playing *Operation* on your face.

After cutting open my pimples, she would then take a device similar to a bobby pin (guess where my wife got the idea from) and would squeeze out all of the blood and white goopy pus balls from the openings. This would cause a lot of bleeding. So much so that she would have to use pressure and healthy dose of gauze to stop it. Sound fun yet? It gets worse.

On top of cutting me open and squeezing the juices out of me, she would proceed to take out every black head she could find. Sometimes they would be next to the fresh scalpel cuts on my face. It was a double whammy of pain. After being tenderized, cut open, and prodded now came the acid baths. She would start by brushing glycolic or salicylic acid on my face. Sometimes she would do both.

If you've ever had that annoying itch after a mosquito bite, then picture that but multiplied exponentially and you may have an idea of what glycolic acid feels like. It was incredibly itchy and I wasn't allowed to scratch my face because it had to soak in. The salicylic acid on the other hand, was more like having a blow torch on your face. That stuff burned! It burned so bad I had to keep myself from getting up and running out of the room. I imagine that's what pepper spray feels like.

Next, came a light water misting that would bring relief from the itching and the burning. She would then drip green minty drops from some kind of medicine on my face. I would walk away looking shiny, smelling minty, and looking bloodied. It was paradise. Obviously, I'm being cynical.

This would happen once or twice a week. My face would look great for about a day or two, but not long after I would explode with more pimples again! The solution was of course to buy more soaps, more creams, and of course maybe we could try some kind of treatment or supplement. All of this was of course futile. No matter what I did, I felt I was cursed to have acne forever. There was no escape.

What gave? Why, no matter what I tried, did the acne not go away? Was it my genes? Was it my lot in life to forever be cursed with these crater making, shame inducing, painful red bulbs on my body?

Before I continue I'd like to point out that the aesthetician and I became good friends during our visits, so I'm not trying to vilify her. The way she approached acne was the same way it's been approached for decades; to look only at the surface of the problem and not consider what's happening in your body at a much deeper level. To her credit, she did recommend I drink more water and avoid greasy foods, though this by itself gave me no incentive to try it more.

If you've ever tried multiple solutions to a problem like acne, then you know how annoying it is to try a system for a long time and have someone tell you it's your fault when it doesn't work. Don't get me wrong. Sometimes we don't fully follow the advice that what we should be when it comes to our health, but what happens when you've done everything you can to fix a problem and it still doesn't work? This issue is more than likely with the system being used and not the person using it.

Typical acne treatments don't address the true, beneath the skin problems that cause acne. If the root cause of acne isn't dealt with, it doesn't matter how many products, pills, soaps, supplements, or creams you throw at it. It will not go away. It will always be taunting you just below the surface ready to pop out in the most embarrassing way at the most inconvenient time. The good news is there's a lot you can do to stop acne that's simple, doesn't require a PhD in science, and actually tastes pretty good. The cause of your acne is food and stress. I'll reiterate that point. Food and stress are the causes of acne. The right foods and a little self-love are all you need as a solution.

The American Academy of Dermatology used to say there is no relation between acne and food [1]. Their position has since started to change.[2] Saying there is no relation between diet and food is a misinformed position [3]. Manufactures of skin care products, repeated that misinformation in the internet and have sold millions of units of soaps and facial creams all while telling people that they can continue to consume foods that can and/or will make acne worse. We'll discuss the kinds of foods that make acne worse later.

The point is, for the last 50 years, there has been overwhelming research that points to food as the leading cause of acne. Study after study has shown that if you eat certain types of foods in excess, or for some people in any amount, you will guarantee and acne outbreak. Some people may experience an outbreak in a few hours to a few days. So what is acne exactly?

---

[1] Bershad SV, "Diet and acne—slim evidence, again, J Am Acad Dermatol (2005);53(6): p. 1102; author reply p. 1103

[2] http://www.aad.org/stories-and-news/news-releases/growing-evidence-suggests-possible-link-between-diet-and-acne

[3] http://www.medscape.com/viewarticle/722953_3

3:
WHY DOES PHAROH HAVE A PIMPLE?

There are several different kinds of acne and they can all happen at the same time on your face. The first two types of acne that you're probably more familiar with are called white heads and black heads.

A white head happens when your pore closes up and swells to a small white dot on your face. These, while annoying, usually don't get too big. Black heads happen when the pore is clogged but still kind of open. The blockage in the pore oxidizes (rusts) and you get a black looking protrusion. You've probably seen some pore strips that are like tape for your face to remove black heads. These strips are good at removing blackheads, but like most treatments they don't get to the root cause.

The next two types of acne that can occur are called pustules and papules. A pustule happens when a white head gets too big and the pore wall breaks underneath the surface of your skin. This type will fill with yellowish pus and can sometimes look like a blister. Papules are hard bumps on your face that don't give very much when you touch them. They can feel like sand paper when you rub your finger over them.

Nodules and Cysts are the type of acne that look really severe and can be very painful. These types of acne go much deeper into the skin and are more prone to scarring. A nodule is usually deep in the surface of the skin and is really hard to the touch. If you've ever tried squeezing one of these to pop it, you've probably discovered that there's no opening for anything to come out. Plus it hurts like crazy. Cysts are soft and pus filled but are still deep below the surface. This is the type of acne that happened to me where the size of the pimple equaled the size of my iris. When my aesthetician friend and I met, this was the first type of pimple she treated. Her treatment worked to get rid of that particular one, but I developed two more cysts in the exact same spot later.

Do any of these seem familiar? Are you experiencing all or some of them? Regardless of the kind of acne you have, it's no less painful. One zit or forty, the only difference is how many of them hurt, not whether or not they do. So when and where did acne make its first appearance? Most people believe it's been around forever. Yes and no. Reports of acne do go all the way back to the Romans, Greeks, and even the Egyptians. What's interesting to note is that the people that got acne were usually those that were better off economically. Most people couldn't afford finer foods like dairy and pastries, so they usually stayed acne free. Those types of foods were reserved for the upper class and the rich. Guess who got acne?

Egyptian writings mention pharos suffering from acne[4]. Must be great to have "the morning and evening star, god on earth" with cysts on his face. Perhaps those pimples were derived from

---

[4] http://johnsern.articlealley.com/the-history-of-acne-223237.html

his magnificent god like eminence. Fun fact: Egyptians thought if someone suffered from acne, then they must be a liar. I'd be curious to see if that applied to the pharos as well.

The Greeks described acne in much detail. Homer and Herodotus mention it in their writings. They really didn't know what to do about it and figured it was contagious. If you had acne back then, it wasn't uncommon for people to avoid you. We now know that acne is not contagious. Kind of sad when the leader of a city state had to be quarantined because people thought he might spread his explosive zits with everyone.

The romans had some success with acne treatments. They were able to mix sulfur with a mineral bath mixture to dry out the skin[5]. It didn't cure acne, but it did help in reducing the redness and oil associated with it. The romans were right about one thing, clogged pores can cause acne. The sulfur mineral bath penetrated the pores, helped unclog them, and helped kill bacteria in the skin.

---

[5] http://www.aqhealth.com/skin-care/acne-treatment/history-of-acne-egyptian-roman-greek-perspective-2300.html

Two thousand years later, humanity's understanding of acne didn't advance much until the early 20th century. Even then few treatments have been truly effective and at best are only for a short while. In the 1930's, benzyl peroxide began to be used to kill bacteria under the skin thus reducing the number of breakouts. Benzyl peroxide, while effective for some people, has little effect for others. This has led to a real problem: the only other real advancements in the treatment of acne have come from more aggressive meds.

Surely something can be done by now. We're supposed to be living in a scientific age of learning and reason where these kinds of things shouldn't be an issue. Science has caught up with the acne question, but just because someone is a scientist doesn't mean they have read the latest research and literature. There are literally thousands of articles related to the treatment of acne without medication and the dangers of using certain medications for prolonged periods of time.

This is probably the chief problem when it comes to a traditional understanding of acne. Dermatologists, MD's and other health

professionals have been so busy trying to treat acne that no one really has time in a literal 16 hour work day to brush up on the latest research showing how to take control of acne. It's the same as trying to swat flies from a pile of poo instead of just getting rid of the pile. Go to the source and you won't have flies. Go to the cause of acne and you won't have breakouts. It's simple. It's time for a healthy dose of truth.

> ### My Acne Nightmare:
>
> *I get acne every time I start stressing. Having to run my store with just 7 employees working 66 hours a week is really stressful while only making $30,000 a year. Trying to hire people is a pain. I get one big red zit on my right cheek or my chin, every time.*
>
> ### Audrey's Story- 23 years old

<u>Part Two:</u>

Acne Misinformation

<u>4</u>:
IS THIS TOOTHPASTE SUPPOSED TO STING?

As long as there has been acne, there have always been remedies. From not touching your face because "you'll make it worse", to putting toothpaste on every pimple and even squeezing lemon juice on your skin, acne remedies are a penny a dozen. Just search on the internet for acne home remedies and enjoy the confusing, contradictory information. One site says don't do this and the other says to do what the other site said not to do. Wait... What? Exactly my point. Sheer and utter confusion.

Typical acne home remedies consist of a little or a lot of the following: alcohol rubs, hydrogen peroxide, toothpaste, lemon juice, popping your own pimples, staying away from Wi-Fi (I wish I was making that up), facial masks made from clay that is found in some obscure jungle or mountain, you name it and it's all but guaranteed to help your pimples.

The problem is that if you've tried any of these things you know firsthand that a lot of them don't work, or if they do they can sometimes cause more damage than they fix.

Let's take toothpaste for example. Toothpaste has been part of the acne home remedy arsenal for years. It's considered a weapon of acne mass destruction for its effectiveness. To apply this remedy, (I'm not recommending you do this at all) take a dab of toothpaste on your finger and place it on the pimple. Massage into your face until you feel a slight burning sensation. Rinse off with cool water and voila. You'll have a reduced acne spot with painful redness and irritation. The point is, this is not a good idea. Some people have tried the toothpaste remedy and wound up with spots from where it was used. Toothpaste is excellent on teeth and for some does reduce their acne. However, the risk of permanently damaging your skin is too high. Let's use toothpaste for what it was intended for- teeth.

Lemon has been used as a remedy as well. The logic is the acid in the lemon juice, and the Vitamin C will reduce or take away the pimple. Admittedly this does work for some people, but do you really want to be putting lemon juice on your face for the years that you have acne? Lemon juice can burn the wound in your face. Picture a mini blow torch on an acne opening and you'll know pain. To be honest with you, I think lemon juice is worse than a scalpel on your face. The acid is very painful. Why must healing always be associated with pain? It shouldn't and it doesn't have to.

Ice has been used to reduce the inflammation of acne. This one is actually a good idea to try if you've got a big pimple that needs to be taken care of sooner than later. With my cystic acne, ice did help bring the inflammation down. It turned the pimple purple, but having a smaller pimple was much better than having a huge one. If you're going to use ice, please understand that it doesn't solve the problem. All it really does is help with the appearance of acne. Nothing more.

Alcohol rubs have been used to help acne, but the major problem with alcohol is that it can leave your skin dry. The fumes can also make you sick. My advice? Stay away from the alcohol rubs. It will kill the bacteria underneath the surface of your skin, but if you're not careful it can lose its potency on your skin due to bacterial resistance.

Masks are used to help people find acne relief and while some work, others spread the acne further over your body. There's a fascinating reason for this that we'll talk more about later. Anyway, be careful with masks. Some people swear by them and others have paid the ultimate facial price for using them; pimples everywhere.

Remedies can't just be dismissed as rubbish or myths, some of them do work. However, thinking of them as miracle cures doesn't solve the problem. If you've ever had a best friend that swears by the toothpaste method then you know what I mean. Take the movie *My Big Fat Greek Wedding*. Tula's father put Windex on every part of his body that was hurting. Her husband even tried it and apparently it took away his pimple. I'm willing to bet some people actually tried it. It may have even worked for some them, but for others it probably burned their faces. If you've ever tried a remedy that worked from someone but not for you, then you know what I'm talking about. Please do not try putting any type of glass cleaner on your face.

Remedies still fail to get to the root cause of acne. They're okay at trying to take the direct approach, but they are only as effective as the depth of skin they penetrate. This is the same problem with topical medications. They can only go so far.

5:
SIDE EFFECTS INCLUDE...DIARRHEA?

Few approaches to acne look at the real cause of acne. Pouring multiple formulations of chemicals on your face or swallowing pills only reduces acne. It never really deals with the source. You can think of it like a firefighter spraying only the flames that are close to him while avoiding the source of the fire in the house. You can keep the flames from getting too far outside the building, but you're not solving the problem. That's why companies are always reformulating their products. They become less and less effective the more and more they're used[6].

Having acne and taking medicine for it are like peanut butter with jelly. The two always go hand in hand, or at least they do in our country. If you've ever searched for acne treatments online, you'll find there are literally thousands of ways to "treat" your acne. Most of them involve some kind of chemical treatment either through a pill or some other means.

The pharmaceutical industry has tried its hand at dealing with acne with varying results. Burned and reddened skin resulting from allergic reactions to creams or masks are not all that uncommon. Lowered ability to fight sickness in addition to scaly skin also happen pretty frequently. Many side effects are worse than the actual disease. Acne meds can also cause a host of other sicknesses that require more meds to fix later, which then cause more things requiring even more meds. It really is a vicious cycle. Some literature shows that prolonged use of benzyl peroxide can lead to

---

[6] http://www.cdc.gov/getsmart/antibiotic-use/antibiotic-resistance-faqs.html#how-bacteria-resist

certain kinds of cancers[7] though admittedly more research needs to be done.

So here are some of the most commonly used medications for acne along with their sordid side effects. Some of them are still used and some of them have been discontinued due to ineffectiveness or were pulled off the market, though their generic equivalent is still being sold.

Isotretinoin (Accutane)-Originally marketed as a chemo therapy drug. Accutane was used to treat acne that did not respond very well to traditional antibiotics. Side effects included birth defects, Irritable Bowel Syndrome, Crone's disease, bone injuries due to thickening/thinning, bleeding or swollen gums, peeling skin, nosebleeds, hair loss, muscle aches, dry skin, dry eyes, slow wound healing, among other things[8]. Accutane went off the market in 2009 due to "economic" reasons as cited by the company[9]. It's also believed that it really had something to do with the overwhelming amount of lawsuits the drug maker Roche was receiving.

---

[7] http://www.ncbi.nlm.nih.gov/pubmed/7784640

[8] http://www.webmd.com/drugs/2/drug-6661/accutane-oral/details#side-effects

[9] http://columbia.legalexaminer.com/fda-prescription-drugs/controversy-ridden-accutane-pulled-from-pharmacy-shelves/

Generic variants of this drug are still being made and are available under the names: Amnesteen, Claravis and Sotret.

Tetracycline-Used to treat respiratory infections, bacterial infections, genital and urinary system infections, acne, skin infections, and stomach ulcers among other uses. Side effects include: upset stomach, diarrhea, itching of the rectum or vagina, sore mouth, redness of the skin (sunburn), and changes in skin color. Here are some serious side effects: severe headache, blurred vision, skin rash, hives, difficulty breathing or swallowing, yellowing of the skin or eyes, itching, dark-colored urine, light-colored bowel movements, loss of appetite, upset stomach, vomiting, stomach pain, extreme tiredness or weakness, confusion, joint stiffness or swelling, unusual bleeding or bruising, decreased urination, pain or discomfort in the mouth, throat sores ,fever or chills[10].

Benzaclin(topical)- Used as a topical agent to keep your pores open by killing the bacteria that

---

[10] http://www.webmd.com/drugs/2/drug-5919-73/tetracycline-oral/tetracycline-oral/details#side-effects

cause acne. Side effects include: dry skin, redness, burning, itching, or skin peeling[11].

Yaz(for women)- Used as a form of birth control and moderate acne control for women who are using birth control, or women in general. It works by combining two hormones to prevent pregnancy and regulate hormones in the body. Side effects include: Nausea, vomiting, headache, bloating, breast tenderness, fluid retention with swelling the in ankles/feet, weight change, vaginal bleeding between periods, or missed/irregular periods. Serious side effects are: blood clots, deep vein thrombosis, pulmonary embolism, stroke, heart attack, sudden shortness of breath, chest/jaw/left arm pain, unusual sweating, confusion, coughing up blood, sudden dizziness, fainting, pain/swelling/warmth in the groin/calf, tingling, weakness, numbness in the arms/legs, unusual headaches, headaches with vision changes, lack of coordination, worsening of migraines, sudden/very severe headaches, slurred speech,

---

[11]http://www.webmd.com/drugs/2/drug-20405/benzaclin-top/details#side-effects

weakness on one side of the body, and partial/complete blindness[12].

These are just four of the many medications that are used to treat acne. It would take another book to list them all. I think you get the point. Are all of these potential side effects really something you should risk enduring? Maybe you'll never have any of the side effects, and maybe you do see clearer skin, but in the long term you're immune system is taking a beating. Now comes issues with drug resistant bacteria.

Here's a scenario. You get a urinary tract infection and it burns like crazy to pee. So you go to the doctor to get meds. Oh wait... you're already on antibiotics. Next, your body takes longer to heal because of the drug resistant bacteria. Your body at that point has now gotten used to the drug you were taking for so long. This requires you to get higher doses which can actually damage your intestinal lining or even give you liver failure. I'm not trying to be overly dramatic.

---

[12] http://www.webmd.com/drugs/2/drug-95358-5115/yaz-28-oral/ethinylestradiol-drospirenone-oral/details#side-effects

These things really do happen to people. There's no way of knowing how your body will react. Even if you underwent a litany of tests to see how your body would potentially react to the medication, you don't really know until you try. To top it all off that kind of testing would easily run into the 10's of thousands of dollars. It's way too expensive for most people. It doesn't make sense to take care of one issue only to cause other long term issues later on life. Acne is not something worth eliminating through traditional channels if it comes at the price of your future and longevity.

My Acne Nightmare:

I had a total forehead outbreak for one year. I had to change my hair style to mask it cause I was a sophmore in high school. I cut bangs to cover my forehead (and acne). I had a horrific outbreak. It was everyday. My dad after 6 months took me to a drug store and found a product that he used as a kid. When I change my moisturizer I still get the occasional pimple, but not like I did when I was in high school.

Alma's Story- 57 years old

<u>Part Three:</u>

But I Like Cookies

6:
ACNE AND DIGESTION

In your gastrointestinal tract you have trillions of bacteria in there, right now. Your body is designed to have more gut bacteria then you have cells in your body. Crazy right? This bacteria in your intestines is actually responsible for helping you stay healthy and have a strong immune system. If you keep killing it off with antibiotics, it can actually damage your immune system and contribute to drug resistant bad bacteria in your body. Remember how some of the side effects of antibiotics include diarrhea? This is because some if not all of the bacteria in

STEPHEN J. RODRIGUEZ

your gut starts dying when you take antibiotics. That's what causes the bowel evacuation.

This is also why nausea happens with some medications. You're body is trying to eject something that is not making it feel well and that it knows is harmful to it. I'm not trying to be gross but that is in effect what is happening. Your body loves you and knows what is poisonous to it. It doesn't make sense to keep forcing feeding your body pills it doesn't want. What's worse is that using antibiotics for a prolonged period of time can actually cause long term neurological damage! Seriously. They do this by inhibiting the beneficial bacteria's ability to synthesize vitamin B12 in your gut[13]. They can also damage your body's ability to absorb that B12. So what is vitamin B12 exactly? Not it's not some kind of alcoholic beverage sold at your local bar.

Vitamin B12 is the vitamin in your body that is responsible for neurological health, blood formation, and metabolism in every cell of your body. It also gives you energy. If you're low on B12 you're going to be low on energy and risk

[13] http://umm.edu/health/medical/altmed/supplement/vitamin-b12-cobalamin

some serious health consequences. If you get nothing else from this book, take a B12 supplement! It's really the only supplement I ever recommend because it's not something your body has readily available. I say again, take B12! You'll feel great when you do and some of you will even feel like you can run around the world. It really can be life changing if you take it. This is why your gut health is so important.

You may not realize this but you wear what's going on inside of your body on your skin and face. If you're gut health is bad, you're going to have bad acne, oily skin, mouth sores, and dry/cracking skin. You'll also have other issues in your body that can potentially include thyroid issues. All of this is can be tied back to your gut health. By taking care of your gut, your entire body is taken care of. Constipation is a major cause of acne also. If the body can't eliminate toxins from your blood stream through your poo, then those toxins will try to come out through your skin. Whether they are pimples, sores, or even boils, your body will do whatever it can to get rid of toxicity. I can't stress this enough, proper digestion is essential. If you're not regularly on the toilet, your health will suffer in more ways than just acne.

Here's a simplified, in a nutshell version of how digestion works. After you take food into your mouth and chew it, your body starts releasing different types of enzymes in your mouth and stomach to dissolve the food and hormones to tell your body what to do with the newly chewed food even before it goes down your esophagus.

Once the food goes down your esophagus, it goes straight into your stomach and gets digested over the course of 2-6 hours depending on how you've treated your body. If you've been abusing yourself intentionally or unintentionally, your stomach will take longer to break down any food you take in.

After that, the food exits the stomach and makes its way into your small intestine through a process called peristalsis. Peristalsis is the involuntary movement of your esophagus, stomach, and intestines that moves food through your body while it's digesting.

While this is happening, your pancreas simultaneously revs up your insulin production, your gall bladder releases bile to break down fats, and your liver gets ready to distribute the nutrients its receiving into the rest of the body. While your food is passing through your small intestine, it gets absorbed by tiny finger-like protrusions coming out of the intestinal wall called villi (vil-ai). The beneficial bacteria we talked about earlier, start releasing their own enzymes and boosting your immune system.

When you give your body whole foods the bacteria in your gut love you and your immune system supports you. When you don't give your body whole foods, the bacteria die and you can become depressed and get sick. What does any of this have to do with acne? Keep in mind your blood is the carrier of all of the minerals, nutrients, and/or junk that your body has absorbed. Every place in your body that has blood vessels will get the ingredients that you've put into your body. This explains the breakout cycle.

This is also how medicine is distributed in your body. Whenever you take a pill, that pill breaks open in your stomach and gets absorbed. That's why pills reduce acne. Your blood takes the chemicals in the pill to every part of your body including your face. If you have acne, and the pill is an antibiotic, it kills the bacteria in your face. The side effect is that it kills every other bacteria, beneficial or not, everywhere else in your body also. This is how you wear your gut health on your face. The chemicals in pills, the junk in food, and the lack of nutrition all contribute to the cause of acne.

After reading this, you've got to wonder why it wouldn't be obvious that what you take into your body affects your health. How can it not? Food builds your cells, affects your mood, and gives you a sense of well-being. Stress will give you acne on your face. Neglecting your gut health will do the same. This is why it is essential to love yourself from the inside out by giving yourself life giving, body nurturing foods. When you give yourself permission to love yourself, only then can you begin to deal with the cookie eating monster within yourself.

7:
THE COOKIE EATING MONSTER WITHIN

Cravings-the boon of dieters. Cravings have a gotten a really bad rap. For a long time cravings were seen as the devil, or at the very least a minion of his demonstrated by a lack of self-discipline in someone. Some cravings are just plain odd. Take for example pregnant women. They have the weirdest cravings in the world! Some of them crave dirt exhibiting a condition called Pica. Others crave pickles and ice cream. Some cravings are for french fries in ice cream, while others get really bizarre.

So what is a craving exactly. A craving is your body's way of telling you what it needs. This is actually key to getting rid of your acne if you do crave certain foods. When your body is missing come kind of nutrient, vitamin, or other type of substance that it needs, it will make you remember a certain kind of food. Just because you remember a certain kind of food though, doesn't mean that particular food you're craving is the best source for what you're missing. Sometimes cravings are actually indicative of something much deeper like an emotional issue.

This can sometimes cause your own personal internal cookie eating monster to rear his cute, ugly head. When I was a kid my mom would occasionally buy pink glazed cookies from the bakery in the town she grew up in. Being 46 miles away meant this really was an occasional treat. I loved those cookies so much. When I grew up, that bakery churned out pink glazed cookies like crazy every Thursday (I memorized the baking schedule). I started to do some part time work there and had the beautiful realization that I could have pink glazed cookies anytime I wanted! It was heaven on Earth...

Every Saturday I would buy a dozen pink glazed cookies on my way out of town and finish every last one of them by the time I got home- 45 minutes later. Occasionally, I would buy an "extra" one for my wife. The problem was she hated them. Even though I knew this, I would still buy it and would of course have to eat it because "I couldn't let it go to waste".

What was the cause of my cookie eating monster's addiction? Was it the sugar in the cookies? In my case, it was actually the stress of the work that I was doing. It was super stressful work. My body was using the cookies as a crutch for both energy and emotional well-being. Kind of sad right? It was a pretty dark time.

Stress is one of the leading causes of acne for several reasons. One of the reasons is that when you're stressed you tend to eat a lot of sugar or other stuff that can cause inflammation in your body. Food becomes a coping mechanism for that stress. You've probably found yourself in front of a tub of ice cream after losing a job, a relationship, or just dealing with day to day stress.

Stress itself releases a potent hormone cocktail that can inflame your acne without food being a contributing factor at all. Stress that goes unanswered will lead to emotional and/or physical starvation. You've got nourish every part of you like anything else. We'll get back to this point in a second.

Take for example sugar cravings. If your body is craving sugar, and we now know sugar makes acne worse, why would your body crave it if it's trying to get rid your acne? Truth be told, you're not actually craving sugar even though your body is telling you, you are. You're actually craving energy! The other possibility is your're looking for comfort from some kind of trauma. Remember ice cream? Your body is missing the necessary components that give it energy and love so it's looking for a quick fix.

This is why cravings tend to be on the unhealthy side of food and why many diets scream at you to be self-disciplined and ignore cravings. Ignoring your cravings is unsustainable. Why not give your body what it's needing so it can heal?

Let's say you're craving a piece of toast. Your body might actually be saying that it's looking for vitamins and minerals. This brings up the subject of enriched foods. An enriched food is a food that has had vitamins and minerals artificially added to it due to those substances being lost in preparation. If you're only getting artificial vitamins from enriched bread, then your body will take the artificial vitamins over no vitamins. However, real vitamins are found in real food. If you give your body whole foods, then you'll start craving those foods because your body found a source of real nutrients and not the fake kind.

This is why cravings are so powerful. If you have ever craved something after eating it, then you know that you're body is screaming at you for nourishment. The only way to truly get rid of your acne is to nourish your body with life giving foods that will heal you. You've got to flush out the toxic mess of chemicals inside of you including the toxic buildup of emotions. If you're feeling emotionally distraught your acne can flare up from that distress. How you deal with these emotions and how you deal with food though, is different from person to person.

8:
BIOLOGICALLY INDIVIDUAL

Individuality is something that we uniquely and consciously hold dear as a species. We're the only species in the world that, as individuals, can change the entire direction of our lives from one day to the next. From the kind of house we live in the climate we thrive in, it's what truly sets us apart from each other. For example, some of us like to go skiing and love cold weather while others of us not so much. Every person has had a unique set of experiences that have shaped their lives and given experience to draw from whenever a decision needs to be made. Sure animals recognize themselves in a mirror, but humanity is the only species that demands its own rights and liberties.

It is this uniqueness, this individuality that allows you to share the same name with someone but nothing else. Even though both of you may carry the same last name, your experiences, DNA, and parental interactions make you your own person. A great example of this is how parents deal with their children. Even though siblings grow up in the same household it doesn't mean that they'll like the same things and act the same way. Take two sisters for example. Both are female, both wore the same clothes in childhood (they are twins after all) and both were given access to the same kinds of experiences from food to faith. One sister loves meat, and the other can't stand it. Genetically identical twins are 100% related, but each one is still a unique individual with their own tastes. Of course some twins are identical in every way, but some are not. It is this uniqueness that is truly a wonderful gift.

Have you considered your ideal health? Your health is unique to you. I don't mean in the sense that you are doomed to a life of disease because you lost the genetic lottery. I mean that you're body has its own unique way of keeping you healthy. When it comes to food, one person's food is another person's poison. Both individuals will react very differently at times. This concept is called "Bio-Individuality".

Joshua Rosenthal, founder of the Institute for Integrative Nutrition, came up with this idea after noticing that individuals reacted to the same foods very differently. For example some people, he noticed, were able to eat nothing but fruits and vegetable and feel perfectly fine. Other people would start to feel sick and weak if they didn't add meat to the mix. The point being that regardless of how "good" a food was, each person's body was going to react to that food the way it wanted to, not the way a one size fits all approach says it should.

I've got a funny/not so funny story for you, a few days before my wife and I found out she was pregnant with our first daughter, I made a wonderful Portobello mushroom steak with rice noodles in peanut sauce. It was divine! She enjoyed it. I enjoyed it and life was great. That is until the middle of the night when the mushroom gods didn't take too kindly to my wife eating one of their own.

My wife woke up and rushed to the bathroom to kneel before that other deity we have a love/hate relationship with: the porcelain god. It all came out in a rush of vomitus glory. She couldn't stand the sight of a mushroom for the next 9 months and to this day, 6 years later, I still can't make that meal without her running from the room disgusted. Are mushrooms bad? No of course not. Mushrooms are full of vitamin D and lots of other nutrients. Her Bio Individual physiology tells her that these particular mushrooms are bad for her. I don't understand why these particular mushrooms prepared this specific way make her sick, but oh well. That's Bio-Individuality at work and I have no interest in poisoning my wife.

So how does this apply to acne? Bio-Individuality is the reason why some people get acne and others don't. It's the reason why some people have giant cysts on their face while other people only have black heads. Rest assured diet and stress are the cause of acne, but Bio-Individuality determines how bad that acne will or will not assert itself not exclusively genetics.

Think about it. Why is it that even in the same family with the same genes, one sibling will have acne only on their foreheads and the other will have it all over their body? This was the case with my brother and me. We both have the same parents, yet my acne was all over my body and my brother's was mainly localized to his face. His stopped at about 22 (he's 34), I still get the occasional small pimple at 28 if I eat too much sugar and dairy. On a side note, whenever I do have a "breakout" it's usually just one pimple as opposed to the massive cysts that would appear on my body when I was younger.

Each person is unique. This is why a one size fits all approach to acne doesn't work. It's why some people can take acne medication and clear up in days while others take that same medication and get on a roller coaster of clear ups and breakouts. It's also why someone can swear by a home remedy and have it work for them, but if someone else tries that remedy it gives them a really bad reaction.

I'm not here to give you a one size fits all approach. On the contrary, my goal is to give you concepts that you can apply in your daily life that are universal. "Wait, I thought you just said you're not shooting for one size fits all. Isn't 'universal' the same thing?" you're probably thinking. No it's not actually. Everyone needs air to breathe. How much air someone can handle depends on the individual. You can't force every person to breathe the same amount of air and expect them al to do equally well. For some people it'll be too much and for others too little. There is no way a child will have the same lung capacity as an Olympic athlete. Basic mathematics has universal concepts that allow you to solve individual problems or really complex ones. You don't need to know every single solution to every problem if you have the concepts to solve them. We're doing the exact same thing. You can take control of your individual acne problem with a tool belt of concepts.

9:
ACNE AND DIET...WHO KNEW?

There are some places in the world that no matter what age you are, whether a teenager, adult or child, acne is nonexistent in the population. They literally have no acne whatsoever. Interestingly enough, they also have no heart attacks, strokes, hardening of the arteries, memory loss, diabetes, dementia, high blood pressure, or obesity among other things, which are a reality of daily life for people in developed countries. One such place is an island off the coast of Papua New Guinea called Kitava[14].

Kitava has been studied for many years by scientists trying to understand why the people are so healthy. These people don't have access to modern medicines, yet they are healthier than most people on the planet. The leading causes of death on the island include, homicide (yikes), pregnancy complications, malaria, accidents, and old age.

These are really healthy people. They have no acne whatsoever. Let's take the developed world on the other hand. If you look at the developed world and developing nations that have adopted a western lifestyle, their rates of acne exploded in their populations.

Is it a genetic thing maybe? Perhaps the Kitavans have developed some sort of genetic immunity to acne, right? The truth is they haven't. They have 46 chromosomes just like you and I do. There is absolutely no genetic difference between them and us other than they're Kitavan and more than likely you and I

---

[14] http://www.staffanlindeberg.com/TheKitavaStudy.html

aren't. They eat food, they sleep, and even use the bathroom! I know, shocking! I'm not trying to be condescending. It's just frustrating how the education systems of the world continually advocate that disease is independent of diet. At the very least, this is a very misinformed approach to understanding acne or any other disease for that matter.

The developed world does a poor job of trying to understand the causes of disease. Take for example, someone that has lived in a country with a more traditional lifestyle. I'm not talking a fast food, microwaved lifestyle. I mean a go out into the field and pick your own food lifestyle.

This person, while living in their home country is usually not obese, has high stamina/energy, and hardly gets sick. What happens when they come to the U.S.? Suddenly they become prone to heart disease, hypertension, diabetes, acne, and a host of other immunological diseases. Why is it that in their home country they don't experience these diseases, but the second they hop on a plane and cross the pond, they start getting sick? Hint: it has absolutely nothing to do with their genes and everything to do with what they started eating once they got here.

I have often joked that there needs to be a thorough investigation and huge studies funded to find out what atmospheric phenomena transforms people's DNA from a robust helix, to the disease prone one they land with at the airport. In truth, their DNA, your DNA, and my DNA are all fine. For the most part the vast majority of us don't have any sort of genetic disorder. Don't get me wrong some people really do have legitimate genetic disorders. All I'm saying is we can't cry wolf when it comes to DNA again and again like we're doing. This idea of genes being the problem causes other problems in and of itself.

Literally 75-90% of teenagers in developed countries suffer or have suffered from some form acne at one point in time or another. Maybe they don't have it constantly bothering them, but they have gotten at least a pimple here and there. Acne seems relentless in trying to embarrass whoever it strikes and does not respect age, career, political office, or anything else.

The United States spends almost $3 trillion on health care every year. You'd think with that kind of budget we would able to make headway in curing acne and other diseases. Yet here we are throwing more money at a problem that many refuse to understand.

As I said before the Kitavans don't suffer from acne period. It's just not in their population[15]. They aren't the only ones either. The Maasai in Africa, assuming they're eating a more traditional diet, don't get acne. The Inuit people in Canada didn't start seeing acne in their population until they started eating a more westernized diet.

Don't get me wrong, a western diet tastes so, so good. But like anything else, just because it tastes good doesn't mean it should be eaten. Dogs lick up anti-freeze on the side of the road, but rest assured it'll kill them within a day. Coincidentally, anti-freeze contains a sugar that lowers its freezing point giving it a sweet flavor. Before I continue DO NOT drink or taste anti-freeze. You run the risk of serious injury or

---

[15] http://archderm.jamanetwork.com/article.aspx?articleid=479093

death. You will die if you drink it. Don't do it. Don't try it.

Funny though how no one questions that drinking poisonous things like anti-freeze will kill you, but food won't do a thing to you. The problem with our food really boils down to this. Our so called "foods" aren't really food at all. I'm referring of course to pre-packaged, boxed foods. They're actually highly chemicalized food derivatives. They aren't real. Read an ingredient label on a bag of chips once in a while and you'll quickly see that there isn't much that comes from the ground or grows on a tree. On a bag of hot and spicy cheese chips you'll find ingredients like: Monosodium Glutamate, Whey Protein Concentrate, and Sodium Diacetate among others.

If all you eat are chemicals, then you won't have any kind of food in your body to build your health or much of anything else. It's like trying to build a house with rotten wood. You need strong wood to put sheet rock on. You need a sturdy foundation to make sure that everything in the house holds up once it's been built. If you build a house out of rotten wood and set it on a poor foundation, don't be surprised when it falls apart because it will. To be honest, it'll be a miracle if it even stays up long enough to put a roof on it. Your body is no different.

Our Standard American Diet, also called a S.A.D. diet is really the problem with acne and disease. It's the root cause of most of our sicknesses. It makes infections linger in the body longer than necessary. It causes your body to break down sooner than later and promotes chronic disease. I can't say this enough. You are what you eat. It's like the car example I gave earlier. The cells in your body are made up of whatever you give them. If you're trying to build a skyscraper out of steel you probably shouldn't be using copper beams. They'll bend with the weight of the structure and the building will collapse. Your body is not that different from that example. I'm not trying to rant about other diseases and go off on a tangent, though I will admit I have come dangerously close. I'm trying to really iterate the fact that food is everything. It literally makes us, or it will break us. The problem with acne boils down to a developed world diet.

With bio-individuality in mind and a western diet taken into account, we need to take a look at foods that make acne worse. Once you understand what makes certain foods so harmful, acne becomes far easier to manage and eliminate. Another nice side effect of using food to foster acne reduction/elimination is a healthier body overall. If you're overweight, you will start taking the pounds off without you even trying. They'll come off even without exercise. I'm not saying don't exercise. I'm saying your body begins to find the balance it's been looking for, but has been unable to find because it didn't have the tools it needed. I'll get to more of that later.

Before I get into the next chapter, I want to stress that I'm not saying you should never eat these foods I'm talking about and going to talk about ever again. What I am saying is that excessive amounts of these foods will cause your acne to flare up like kerosene in a fire.

10:
IF YOU WANT AN OUTBREAK, EAT THIS

Refined sugar, or any food item that turns into a sugar when it hits your bloodstream is the first kind of food that makes acne worse. So what kinds of foods fall into this category? Well, there are some obvious culprits. Sugary sodas are a big candidate for causing acne flare ups. This is because the bacteria in your pores feeds on the sugar in these drinks and causes an infection. As a matter of fact, some scientists have started experimenting with using sugar as a delivery vehicle for medicines in treating bacterial infections. Thank you drug resistant bacteria.

Turns out bacteria has lost its appetite for antibiotics. Whenever these drug resistant bacteria "see" an antibiotic coming at them, they shut down their metabolism and go into hibernation. They won't even touch the antibiotics because somehow they now "know" that it'll kill them. They, like all living organisms, want to survive and multiply. They don't want to die. Apparently bacteria are smart enough to know not to "eat" certain kinds of chemicals. They don't have brains so what's really happening here? To be honest, this phenomena is not understood very well by science yet so I can't really give you an answer. What can be said doesn't go beyond the obvious, "Wow this is fascinating. We need to learn more about this."

The new approach to killing these bacteria is to hide antibiotics in sugar so the bacteria will eat the sugar antibiotic mixture and die[16]. I think we're missing the point here. If bacteria loves sugar so much, why aren't dermatologists recommending that acne sufferers get off of sugar? I can say with certainty that you're

---

[16] http://healthland.time.com/2011/05/16/could-a-spoonful-of-sugar-help-the-medicine-work/

probably not eating sugar with antibiotics in it. When any living organism eats something that is good for it, it grows and continues with the processes of its life. Bacteria, while small and not easily visible, do exactly that but in your pores. Sugar makes bacteria grow.

It's the reason why if you are sick with an infection, sugary drinks or anything with sugar in general will make that infection worse. At the very least it will keep the infection around longer. It's the reason why antibiotics are becoming less and less effective at controlling any kind of infection, let alone acne. Natural sugars like those found in fruit and fruit juices are different though. They don't react the same way with bacteria. Natural juices such as orange, apple, or grape juice etc. don't cause acne flair ups, or typically make infections worse. This is because they are not refined. You're drinking them the way nature packaged them. Now if you see a juice bottle that says 100% juice from concentrate, these juices can and most likely will make acne worse. The reason being is even though the label says 100% juice, usually manufacturers will add some kind of refined sugar anyway to help it taste better and "preserve" it.

When a natural sugar is refined, whether it be sugar cane or something else, most if not all of its whole foods natural goodness is lost to the refinement process. The anti-oxidants, fiber, vitamins and minerals are all stripped from the original product with almost none of them left behind. All that's left over is a crystal granule that looks nothing like the original sugar. This causes other health problems with acne and other areas of your body.

Sugar is also pro-inflammatory[17]. If you have a red, swollen, and/or hot tender area in any place on your body, that's called inflammation. That's exactly what acne is. It's a red, swollen, and warm tender area of skin on your face. Refined sugar promotes inflammation. The fact is that your body was not meant to consume refined sugar in the excessive amounts that most people do.

Did you know that in one 20 oz. soft drink bottle, the amount of sugar inside that bottle will

---

[17] http://ajcn.nutrition.org/content/94/2/479.long

fill up 1/3 of the bottle? Think about that. If you were to take all of the liquid out of the soft drink, you would have a small mountain of sugar inside that bottle. Never mind the amount of sugar in 3 liter bottle. How many 3 liters bottles of a soft drink have you had in the last month, the last week or the last few days? If you drink a soft drink with every meal the problem is only multiplied.

If you think artificial sweeteners may be the answer, bad news. There's new evidence that may show artificial sweeteners are allowing blood sugar levels to spike and cause potential breakouts. Admittedly, this evidence is not well understood, but the possibility of artificial sweeteners contributing to acne is not out of the realm of possibility.

You're probably mad at me right now for taking all of the fun out of life. I'm not trying to do that. I stress again. I'm not saying don't ever eat sugar, I am advocating a balanced life style that promotes health and wellness as a way to get rid of your acne, or at the very least bring it under control.

My Acne Nightmare:

When I was in middle school I had acne all over my neck. It was very embarrassing. I would eat a lot of junk food and get big break out afterwards. I'm talking about my entire neck. All over.

Matt's Story- 29 years old

Candy bars and hard candies also fall into the category of refined sugar. Curiously enough, candy bars contain milk chocolate giving you a double whammy of dairy and sugar. This is why the old wives tale says that chocolate causes acne. It's not the chocolate that's causing acne, it's actually the milk and sugar in the chocolate that's contributing to acne formation.

Even though some people eat milk chocolate and don't get breakouts, for other people, milk chocolate is a like an acne switch. They will get a massive breakout. This is why Bio-Individuality is important. Everyone is unique. Each person has a different acne trigger. Yours will not be the same as someone else's though it might be similar.

White breads and enriched grains also cause problems for people with acne. These "grains" are actually stripped of all their nutritional value and are "enriched" with artificial vitamins and minerals to replace what was taken out. Basically they're like insta-sugar. They turn to sugar almost immediately once they enter the stomach and get into your body. Sugar=inflammation. Inflammation=bad acne.

All acne is, is a symptom of the greater inflammation happening in your body. Your body is telling you on your face, that there is something much deeper happening inside of you. It's why acne medications try to penetrate deeply into the pore, or are taken by mouth to work from the inside out. If you had a problem with a tree growing incorrectly, and you replaced it with another tree. If that new tree grew incorrectly as well, it doesn't make sense to keep pulling the trees out, or to try and give them tree medicine to make them better. The problem is something in the soil or the soil itself.

Acne is your body's way of saying, "There is something wrong with me". Internally the environment in your body is allowing acne to flourish and thrive. By putting refined sugars in your body, you're actually ensuring that acne will be around for a long time. Sugar has to become persona non grata in your body when it comes to acne. That's Latin for an unwelcome person.

So to summarize what you just learned, sugar causes inflammation and feeds the bacteria under your skin giving you a giant infected mound on your face, but sugar isn't only found in candy bars, bread, and drinks. It can also be found in milk. While we've already established that too much sugar is bad, milk has some other problems with it. "What!?! No! How can you be attacking dairy?" you ask. Let's do a quick anatomy lesson.

Acne is thought to form when the sebaceous glands in your pores produce too much oil. The oil then traps dead skin cells clogging your pores and allowing bacteria on your face to infect those pores. The result is a pimple whether giant or small. Cystic acne happens when that process gets really bad and happens deeper into the skin. We talked about that in the beginning. That pimple I told you about that was the size of the iris in my eye, was a cyst.

What does dairy have to do with this? Turns out the sebaceous glands respond to hormones in your body. Hormones are like the chemical keys inside your body. Just like a keyhole on a door, hormones tell your cells to do certain things and react certain ways. Your sebaceous glands respond to hormonal changes in your body and either produce more or less oil depending on the load of hormones their getting.

Milk and other dairy foods are actually full of additional hormones that don't go away during pasteurization. Hormones like Insulin-like Growth Factor One (IGF-1) and Recombinant Bovine Growth Hormone (rBGH). This means that if you're a teenager and your hormones are already out of control, then you're adding a ton of additional hormones into your body that it doesn't need[18]. Your body responds by having acne pop out all over you like a glorified game of Whack-A-Mole. If

---

[18] http://www.ncbi.nlm.nih.gov/pubmed/15692464

you're an adult, it means that the hormonal balance that you worked so hard to achieve during puberty is now being thrown completely off. Some adults experience chronic acne well into their 30's and 40's.

I used to have acne all over my face, head, neck, back, chest, and arms. I would get the occasional pimple on my foot or leg as well. If you've ever experienced this, there is nothing more annoying in my opinion than a pimple inside your nose. Foods like milk and cereal don't help bring acne under control either. That's right! The breakfast of champions that is supposedly part of balanced breakfast may actually be throwing your body's hormonal balance off.

It's not just limited to teenagers though. Women that go through their menstrual cycles due to the intense hormone fluctuations in their bodies, will either have acne come out or get worse due to excessive dairy consumption and eating foods that contain additional hormones. Men are equally susceptible to acne. If a man decides to take hormonal supplements or he begins to exercise more, he will have a tendency to get more acne on his body. The reason for this is twofold.

First the sweat on his brow may become bacteria food. If his immune system is already weakened and he's already internally inflamed like we've talked about before, then acne is all but guaranteed. Couple that with the fact that he's probably going to have some kind of meat based protein and possibly milk to "build strong bones"; more than likely acne will soon be on its way. That hot body he was looking forward to showing off to the ladies, will now have red oily masses on his face.

The point is, if you eat sugary foods and consume a lot of dairy, then you are painting mini targets on your face in the form of acne and you don't even know it. According to the FDA (The U.S. Food and Drug Administration), milk does not cause acne. This is gross misinformation. To support their claim, they argue that pasteurization, the process that we use to sterilize certain foods, burns out 90% of the hormones in milk and that the rest of the hormones are taken care of in your stomach through digestion. Therefore, acne is not a possible outcome with milk consumption because there aren't any additional hormones going into the body.

The problem with their argument lies in how they demonstrated this "no hormone in milk" effect. Traditional pasteurization heats milk up to 162 degrees Fahrenheit for 15 seconds in order to kill any germs that might wind up in the bottling process.

The FDA used a study that heated the milk to 162 degrees Fahrenheit for 30 minutes. Did you catch that? They didn't use the same amount of time as traditional pasteurization. They used 28 minutes and 45 seconds more time than required. When they heated up the milk this way, that's when they got a 90% reduction in the hormones in milk. What they didn't say was that when milk was heated for 15 seconds, not 30 minutes, then only 19% of the hormones were "burned" out of the milk. This means that 81% of the hormones in milk that leave the cow go into your body when you drink it[19].

---

[19] http://articles.mercola.com/sites/articles/archive/2008/01/02/dairy-industry-self-destructs.aspx

Since acne is directly related to the hormone load in your body, drinking milk and eating dairy makes acne worse! Let's look at some examples. Whenever my wife eats too much dairy, she'll have a mini breakout. You're probably saying, "Your wife hardly constitutes the population at large." That's true, but if you have acne ask yourself this, "Do I eat or drink a lot of dairy?" and, "Do I drink enough water?" If the answer to those questions are yes and no respectively, then you probably need to make some changes. If I have too much dairy, the same thing happens to me.

By the way, my breakfast of choice almost every morning growing up was milk and cereal. I now have the scars on my face from that choice. It bothered me most when my 4 year old daughter walked up and asked me what happened to my face. It hurt even more when she took her little hand touched my cheeks because she though my face still hurt. This is not something you want to continue.

Once again, I'm not saying you can never drink anything except water, or that you can never drink milk ever again. What I'm saying is that you're probably having too much dairy and not enough water so your body has no choice but to react with acne. Try cutting back on dairy, or if you can, stop it altogether and watch the acne disappear right off your face.

Refined sugars and milk aren't the only types of food that make acne worse. Meats can be just as harmful. Let's talk about farms for a second. Whenever someone mentions a farm with animals, what's the first image that comes to mind? Is it Bessie grazing in a field with her calf as farmer Bill is riding his tractor collecting hay? Perhaps you imagine a lot of mooing and frolicking. While this is a pretty rosy picture of livestock farms, the reality is actually far darker.

Cow farms, where we get our meat from, are actually pretty gross places for any living thing. I'm not going to go on a vegan rant about how bad it is to eat animals. I'm not vegan. I am going to be very factual though about what happens out there.

First of all, the cows are not in grassy fields that are green and rosy. They're usually standing in mud or poop all day long and are fed from a trough. Instead of giving the cow a diet of grass like its built for, it's given a diet of grain.

This causes some big problems for the cow like death and disease. As a result, the vet has to come in and pump the cow full of antibiotics in order to kill infections. If the cow does survive, it's then given hormone pills to help it grow bigger, faster.

The hormones in these pills are hormones like: estradiol, testosterone, progesterone, androgen trenbolone acetate, and progestin melengestrol acetate[20]. Those are a mouthful I know. The problem is these hormones don't fully cook out of the meat when it's consumed.

All of these hormones affect your body when you're eating a lot of meat. Just like the hormones in dairy cause the sebaceous glands in your face to over produce sebum, the hormones in meat aren't helping either. If your daily meal plan consists of milk and cereal in the morning, a burger for lunch, and a steak for dinner, then no wonder why your acne is out of control. There is no way to tame it. Your body is already on hormonal overload.

---

[20] http://www.organicconsumers.org/articles/article_5543.cfm

Chicken may be a possible culprit in promoting antibiotic resistance[21]. Chickens are given antibiotics and hormones to stimulate growth by killing the bacteria in the gut of the chicken that is supposed to be there. The chicken then has a weakened immune system and is unable to fight off infections. Some antibiotics and chemicals don't cook out of the chicken and go into your body when you eat it. Infections then become harder to kill off for some people.

Throw in refined sugars, and it's actually surprising that your acne isn't worse. In order to reduce/eliminate acne, meat consumption needs to be reduced. I emphasize, I'm not saying never eat meat again. I'm saying reduce it and crowd it out with better foods. Try leaner meats. The next chapter will go into this in more detail. This is really important! If you do decided to stop eating meat, take a Vitamin B12 supplement.

Acne is not an accident. It's the result of an overtaxed immune system responding to a toxic internal environment. We need to reset that

---

[21] http://www.ncbi.nlm.nih.gov/pmc/articles/PMC1257574/

environment in order to promote good skin health. The good news is that's not hard to do. The bad news is, you're probably not going to be able to eat excessive amounts of foods that harm your body. Wait...I think that's good news.

STEPHEN J. RODRIGUEZ

<u>Part Four:</u>

Acne Eradication

11:
I'M AN ADULT. WHY DO I STILL HAVE ACNE?!?

If you're like millions of people who suffer from acne, and you're an adult, you're probably wondering why acne didn't stop in your teenage years. Most of us were told that acne would only be a problem up until we turned 20, then after that something magical would happen and acne would no longer be a problem. By my account, things didn't exactly happen that way. Remember the genetics rant?

I still get the occasional pimple. Thank God it's not as bad as it used to be, but it does still happen. As a matter of fact as of the time of this writing, I just got my first arm pimple in a long time. It's been a crazy week for me. I've done a lot of traveling and unfortunately, Starbucks and I became reacquainted. As you're going to find out and as we've already discussed, you can probably guess why I get the occasional pimple. The answer is really quite simple. I don't follow my own advice sometimes. I'm ashamed to say it, but it's true. I'm just as human as you are.

See, people that write books like this sometimes try to make themselves look like to you, the reader, that they've got all the answers and that they never struggle with the issue that they're writing about in their book. I'm not going to lie to you like that.

I'm really wanting to get everything out in the open so all of us in the developed world can finally have a civil dialogue aimed at getting to the truth of how to get rid of and gain control of acne once and for all. Not every piece of advice in this book will apply to you. Each person has their own Bio-Individuality. However, the good news is the advice and ideas mentioned in this book will clear up acne for the majority.

So here are two things you can do that will set a solid foundation for acne reduction and elimination. They're super easy, and don't require you to do anything special other than what you're doing now. One of the things you can do is so easy. I can tell you with all certainty that you will never forget to do it at least once a day. So no worries.

Remember how we talked about all of the hormones that are inside of food and how those hormones are causing breakouts? Turns out food isn't the only place you'll find hormones. The cosmetics industry actually puts hormones inside of their products all of the time.

If you're a guy reading this then you're probably telling yourself you've got nothing to worry about. Actually you do. So do you ladies. The cosmetics I'm referring to are actually facial creams and shampoos. Makeups and other cosmetics contain petroleum by-products like dyes, clays, and other harmful substances[22] [23]. Remember, your pores are a two way street. Well imagine bathing your face with gasoline. Now I realize that makeup isn't pure gasoline. If

---

[22] http://www.scientificamerican.com/article/where-does-blue-food-dye/

[23] http://www.fda.gov/Cosmetics/Labeling/IngredientNames/ucm109084.htm

it was then you would have burned your face and eyes a long time ago and wound scarred and blind, but some ingredients in makeup come from the exact same oil fields. The way we get petroleum by- products, like those found in makeup and food dyes, is simple and straightforward process.

First the crude oil is trucked or piped in from an oil well. The crude then gets put into a container that's fed into a boiler. The boiler then pipes everything into a giant silo-like tube called a distillation column. Depending on how the oil cools, different by-products float toward the top of the silo and get fed out of different pipes based on their boiling point[24]. Makeups and other cosmetics use some of these by-products in their formulations. The result is you're quite literally putting really old dead things on your face. That's what oil is; a bunch of dead plants and animals that turned to goop far beneath the surface of the earth after a long time and a lot of pressure. It doesn't stop there though.

---

[24] http://science.howstuffworks.com/environmental/energy/oil-refining2.htm

In Europe there are 1,373 chemicals banned in cosmetics[25]. In the United States there are only nine chemicals that are banned for use in cosmetics[26]. Cosmetic companies aren't required to label all the ingredients that go into them. Ingredients like formaldehyde, triclosan, parabens, ethylene oxide and yes, even lead are used all of the time. The FDA, that is the Food and Drug Administration for the United States, has stated that cosmetics companies can use almost *any* ingredients they want to in the manufacturing of their products. Cosmetics companies are also not required to demonstrate the safety of their products. So what does this mean for you? It means, you don't really know what kind of chemicals are going on your face or your body, or what kind of harm they could be doing to you beyond acne.

Triclosan has been found to affect the system in your body that regulates hormones, particularly your thyroid hormone and it can affect reproductive hormones[27]. It's also been found to act like an estrogen mimic in low doses

---

[25]http://ec.europa.eu/consumers/cosmetics/cosing/index.cfm?fuseaction=search.res ults&annex_v2=II&search

[26]http://www.fda.gov/iceci/inspections/inspectionguides/ucm074952.htm

[27] http://www.ncbi.nlm.nih.gov/pubmed/16922622

and has been found in breast cancer tumors. Speaking of breast cancer tumors, parabens have also been found in breast cancer tumors as well. Ethylene oxide is a recognized carcinogen as well formaldehyde. Lead is a neurotoxin and can cause severe neurological damage in humans. Forgive this rant, but watching what goes in and out of our bodies is so important for more things other than our acne.

Triclosan is found in soaps, deodorants, and toothpaste. A recent study that was done found that Triclosan was found to be safe in toothpaste. Whether it really is or isn't remains to be seen. If you're using a lot of different kinds of soaps not really knowing what's in them, there is a possibility that Triclosan may be causing problems with your acne and other places in your body.

It can make for a very frustrating situation. If you're a woman that has a lot of acne and you use makeup to cover it up, you may actually be inadvertently making the problem worse depending on the ingredients that are in your makeup. If you're a guy that is trying to get rid of his acne, the soap you're using may be helping acne to stay. Couple that with hormone laced foods and antibiotic resistance, and you've almost got the perfect storm for more problems beyond acne.

The FDA allows up to 5mg/oz. of progestin to be added to facial creams and shampoos without having to put anything on the label[28]. This means that not only are you potentially getting a hormone overload from your food, but you're also getting doused with hormones every time you put shampoo in your hair. Unfortunately, because many shampoo companies don't label their products, I can't really give you a list of offenders.

Progestin, otherwise known as progesterone in its non-synthetic form, is a hormone that regulates ovulation in women and helps maintain pregnancy. Congratulations men. If you're using a shampoo with progestin in it, then you're on your way to ovulating. I'm kidding, but if you do shampoo every day, then you are getting a constant does of this stuff and it does not bode well for your overall health or your acne.

---

[28] http://www.fda.gov/iceci/inspections/inspectionguides/ucm074952.htm

My Acne Nightmare:

I started getting acne in 7th grade. One minute I was clear and the next I broke out. Went to a dermatologist and tried everything in the world, nothing worked. A cream I would use that the dermatologist gave me made me look like I had a sunburn. It burned my face. I'd get some ingrown pimples in my nose, and the dermatologist would inject it and it would go away the same day. I'd still get them back every so often. For a while they told me it was cause I was eating too much chocolate and coke. That didn't help when I stopped. I drank a lot of milk growing up and still do. At 44 years old man I'm still getting zits. It's ridiculous.

Joe's Story- 44 years old

Ladies, if you've ever noticed a spike in acne around your cycle, your shampoo isn't helping. As for both men and women, if you're using facial creams to help calm acne or moisturize your skin, then you're actually giving your body another dose of progestin. Your facial cream might actually be causing your acne. When you read "Deya's" story toward the end of this chapter, it may have been the reason why she experienced her outbreak when she was trying an avocado mask.

Because the FDA doesn't require cosmetics companies to label their products with an ingredient list, it's a crapshoot as to what you are getting inside of your shampoo. This is where things get a little tricky, because obviously you need to bathe.

The best advice I can give you is to Google what shampoos, creams and additional cosmetics contain hormonal additives. You'll be able to see who adds what to their products and you may even find some products that are hormone free.

If you've ever wondered why acne continued into adulthood for you, this is one of the many reasons why. If you're a teenager, doing nothing will mean that acne will follow you far longer than you'd like. Just like the example of the job interview you read earlier, people will continue to judge. It's not right that they do, but it is the way things are.

Acne doesn't respect age. Even some senior citizens still get acne. It can literally strike at any time. Acne is the combination of a perfect repeatable storm that keeps happening in your life. You need an umbrella. You're probably still going to get a little wet, but it will be nothing compared to the torrential down pour you'll experience through inaction.

So how do you stop the outbreaks from happening if you've done everything to the surface of your skin that you can? How can you take control of your acne for good, and not have to be plagued by it for the rest of your life in some cases?

My Acne Nightmare:

In high school I broke out during the first semester of senior year. I tried everything. I tried an avocado mask and it spread from forehead to the sides of my face. I would get them on my nose. I tried a mask with egg white and lemon that was supposed to clean my face. It didn't work. I tried so many things and finally I tried a mint julep mask. It helped and it finally stopped after I found that. I think it was stress related. You know senior year. You're not sure if you're going to graduate or not. The day before my wedding I was so stressed I had a breakout of about 3 pimples lining my lip. I looked horrible. The lady that was doing my makeup had to cover it up on my forehead and mouth. It still happens when I get behind on my menstrual cycle. I'll breakout on my mouth.

Deya's Story- 24 years old

STEPHEN J. RODRIGUEZ

12:
KEEP IT CLEAN

When it comes to acne, there are a ton of different opinions on what good acne hygiene looks like. Should you wash your face? Should you not wash your face? Should you rub some kind of cream or get a steam facial? The fact is that people do see acne reduction/elimination with these and other things.

To be honest with you, most if not all of these things are great things to do. My whole rant is that you would not rely on them solely. We need to take a holistic approach when it comes to acne. What does holistic mean? It means taking all parts of the person into consideration when dealing with a problem like acne. Not just bacteria, size/type of pimples, and age. The entire person has to be considered when looking at what kind of damage acne is doing to them.

Consider the problem with fast food face a.k.a. fried food face. This particular affliction happens when people work at fast food restaurants frying foods all day. These people usually get really bad acne. They may or may not have a great diet, but all of that oil that's evaporating and latching on to their skin is acting as a bacteria feeding pore clogging mixture, that's all but ensuring scarred skin for the rest of their lives.

These people really need to be washing and cleansing their faces in addition to cleansing the inside of their bodies. If these people don't do BOTH, then the toxicity of the environment that they're in will overtake their immune system and they won't be able to keep acne at bay for long. Cleansing one's face after work when you're frying food all day is absolutely vital.

So what do you do to cleanse your face after

finding out that there are so many harmful ingredients in cosmetic products? Well, I have good news for you. There is an organization in Nova Scotia Canada called The Environmental Health Association of Nova Scotia that has a wonderful website full of alternatives to chemical laced cosmetics products. You can find their website at http://lesstoxicguide.ca. Their website is a great resource where you can find so many great alternatives to harmful products.

What most people don't realize about pores is that they are a two way street. Your pores are used by your body to both absorb and take in substances. This is why pimples swell from the inside out. You're body can't get rid of the toxin/bacteria combination underneath so it tries to push it through to the surface. Total two way street.

If you have ever swam in a swimming pool that was recently cleaned you may have experienced swimming pool face. Swimming pool face is the exact opposite of fast food face. Depending on how long you've been swimming, the chlorine in the water penetrates your pores. The result is clear skin for a day or two. Don't go rubbing chlorine on your face as a means of getting rid of your acne. Pure chlorine is absolutely deadly and will cause you to experience life threatening breathing problems if you come into prolonged contact with it. You will wind up in the hospital and die. The amount of chlorine in a swimming pool isn't concentrated enough to hurt you and has been diluted in the swimming pool's water. This is why it's safe to swim in a chlorinated pool.

My Acne Nightmare:

I was a football player and I had acne really because of the helmet, especially on the chin strap and my forehead. As I got older, it just kept coming. I tried Proactiv. That stopped it for just a few months and it started coming back. I tried oatmeal soap and that really helps. I still get it occasionally

Anthony's Story- 29 years old

It's also why something as simple as washing your pillow will keep acne at bay and be real game changer for a lot of people. When was the last time you heard a dermatologist recommend a pillow washing? Hint: they usually don't.

Imagine if you were lying down on pile of dirt that had been used by animals for a potty (sorry for the terminology, I still have little ones). Now further imagine that you did this every day for at least 6 hours. How much bacteria would you be lying in? Pretty gross right? This is basically the equivalent of sleeping on an unwashed pillow and pillowcase. Every night for at least 6 hours or more you are lying on a bacteria farm that's full of body soil, dirt, and dead skin cells. Let's not forget the mites also. They've got to eliminate waste as well.

The simple act of washing your pillow and your sheets will not only give you clearer skin all over your body, but it will also give you a fresh clean feeling every time you get into bed. Oh by the way, in order to cut down on body soil, you'll probably want to shower every night before bed if possible. This will help keep your sheets fresh, keep the bacteria farms from flourishing, and provide you with a good night's rest. You will sleep much better when the sheets aren't sticking to you.

Sunblock and makeup are notorious pore cloggers. Sunblock, for example, is designed to stay on and be hard to remove without some effort. The idea is to keep you protected from damaging UV sun rays and keep your skin from getting skin cancer while you're at the beach. The downside is that you may have a breakout after wearing sunblock for a long period of time. As with the individual with fast food face, you'll need to get sunblock off as soon as humanly possible to reduce the risk of a breakout.

Makeup is REALLY bad for your skin unless it's been specifically formulated for being gentle on it. I know it's wise and prudent not to fork over a ton of dough for something that costs twice as much for the same product in two different stores, but all makeup is not created equally. Get make up off as soon as possible and if you can't afford the safe kind, then please use it sparingly.

Acne hygiene and personal hygiene above the surface are important, but taking care of what's going on below the surface, deep inside of you, is in some cases far more important. Actually it is more important. Your body uses your skin like your mouth and rectum; as a means of waste removal. Washing the outside cleans what's at the surface but if you're polluted inside, it will come out from within.

In the next chapter we're going talk about several things you can do to reduce if not eliminate your acne in as little as seven days, and keep it off. Are you willing to try?

13:
ACNE ANNIHILATION

Concerning food, there are two things that you can start doing today, that will set the foundation for lasting relief from your acne. You're probably doing one or both of them right now and you don't even realize it. If you're doing these two things already, then why is your acne still so bad? You're probably getting in your own way by stopping them from working by polluting your body, or you're not letting them fully work. I call them the "2 Do's". These "2 Do's" set the foundation. Do them and you your skin will love you.

The first thing you need to do to start reducing and/or eliminating your acne is to drink more...Water! Wait, what? Yep drink more water. You're probably yelling at me right now while you're reading this. You're probably saying, "I do drink water!" More than likely you do drink water, or at least I hope you do. The problem is you probably don't drink enough of it. Ever needed a moisturizer for your face because it was cracked and dry? What about other parts of your skin? Assuming you're not taking a ton of other medications that dry out your skin then guess what? You're not drinking enough water.

Water is an amazing substance-two hydrogens bonded to one oxygen. It's what sustains life on this planet and without it, Earth would be a dead world. Your body is 70% water, or at least it's supposed to be. Most people don't drink anywhere near the amount of water they need to be healthy regardless of whether or not they live in a third world country. So how much is enough? There's no real set amount. I'm not going to confuse you with formulas that show you how much to drink according to your body weight, or how many cups are enough based on your height. It would be pointless to do that. I'm going to make it much simpler. Try drinking a gallon a day. At least that. If you start to feel woozy when drinking water, that's when you're probably drinking too much and you should stop and drink more, later. Your body will let you know. Most people, as in the vast majority, will probably never get to the point of nausea.

Why? Because the beverage of choice for people is usually sugary drinks in some form or another. These drinks are actually making acne worse! (We've talked about this before). By drinking more water, you're reducing the inflammation in your body and laying a foundation for your acne to heal.

Acne, at a basic level, is really just inflammation on your face. Water reduces inflammation. It's that simple. Just to warn you though, you're probably going to be peeing like crazy for a little while. Your body goes into cleanse mode when it starts getting more water and begins to gently detox. Side effects of drinking more water include: temporary frequent urination, smoother skin, less oil/redness in your face, cleaner kidneys, and better circulation and blood flow just to name a few. In other words, your body is going to start getting better in more areas than your face.

Someone asked me once about water toxicity. They heard that if you drink too much water, you can actually get water poisoning. Just to calm any fears, the only real way you can get water poisoning is if you don't pee when your body says to. Tragically a young 28-year old mother died in 2007 after taking part in a radio contest called "Hold you wee for (Nintendo) Wii"[29]. She, along with other contestants, were given bottles and bottles of water to drink without being allowed to urinate, otherwise they would forfeit the prize. The DJ's even joked that she looked 3 months pregnant after having a very swollen belly. She passed away from water toxicity later on that day.

Water toxicity occurs when you don't listen to your body. Many of the contestants complained that they started to feel physically uncomfortable after a while of not urinating and drinking so much. If you hold in your pee then you're more than likely going to feel sick.

---

[29] http://www.nbcnews.com/id/16614865/ns/us_news-life/t/woman-dies-after-water-drinking-contest/

Obviously if you don't urinate at all, your body will respond with extreme illness and death. Drink lots of water, be sure to urinate, and you'll be just fine. If you have deep dark circles underneath your eyes, those will actually start going away also. The rest of your body will have naturally hydrated skin from within, instead of having to put on a ton moisturizers on the outside hoping to lock in some moisture.

This brings us to our next concept called "Crowding Out". Crowding out harmful foods and eating foods that reduce/eliminate acne actually go hand in hand. Remember how in the last chapter I mentioned that I wasn't telling you to never eat foods like milk and cereal, meat, and refined foods again? This is why. If you can eat less of those foods by crowding them out with more good whole foods, then your body will start to heal itself and your acne will go away.

So what kinds of foods heal acne? In a short answer, leafy greens and fruits. Leafy greens? What's that? Hopefully you know what fruit is. Before you get grossed out if you know what leafy greens are, I'm not talking about eating straight kale and broccoli unless you're into that sort of thing. I mean having wonderful nourishing foods that reduce inflammation, give you energy, heal your acne, and give you smooth as a baby's butt skin.

Smoothies are one way to really get your body the jolt of leafy fruity goodness it needs. As a matter of fact, here is a really easy recipe you can use to get started. It takes about 5 to 10 minutes to make and can even act as a meal replacement. You can also find a few other recipes in the back of the book to give you some meal and snack ideas.

A nice side effect of these types of smoothies is that if you're having constipation issues, it'll actually get the pipes running like they're supposed to be. A word of warning though if you've been constipated recently, or you don't go poo every day, you may experience an immediate bowel evacuation. It doesn't mean the smoothie made you sick, it means that you're body has been trying to get rid of that junk in your intestines for a long time and it was finally able to "eject" it.

The reason for this is a thing called fiber. Fiber comes in two forms in plants. One form is called soluble fiber and the other is non-soluble.

Soluble fiber dissolves in the water that's in your body and is absorbed by your intestines. It also helps you feel full if you're eating vegetables in a meal. Non-soluble fiber, doesn't dissolve and acts like an internal bulldozer to push waste out of your body. Fiber is essential to a healthy body whether you're dealing with acne or not. So without further ado here is the recipe:

Green Smoothie Inspired by Vitamix

Ingredients:

Around 1/2 cup of coconut water or regular water (your choice)

1/2 cup of pineapple juice

1/2 of a pear or apple

1/2 cup of spinach leaves (not the frozen kind)

1 broccoli floret

1/2 an avocado

1-2 cups of green grapes.

1 cup of ice

Tools:

Cutting Board

Knife

Blender

To Make The Smoothie:

Chop all of the grapes, broccoli floret, pear/apple into small pieces.

Pour the water and juice into the blender.

Cut the avocado in half and put that half in the blender making sure to leave out the peel.

Pour the grapes, broccoli, and pear/apple into the blender.

Add the ice and start the blender on the ice crushing setting for about 40 seconds or until a smooth consistency is achieved.

Enjoy!

That's pretty much it. Foods like this smoothie promote your body's natural ability to heal itself. They also boost your immune system and help eliminate any other infection you may be dealing with. The bacteria in your gut will love you for this. You are supposed to have more bacteria in your intestines than you do cells in your body. The bacteria, also called flora, are an essential part of your immune system. Without them, you will get sick and have greater difficulty fighting off infections. By the way, on a quick side note, eating fermented foods will actually boost the flora in your gut and aid in digestion also. Cool, huh? It's great. We're not really going to cover fermented foods in this book, but you're welcome to look them up. Yogurt, while being dairy, doesn't seem to react to acne the same way that milk does. Try it and see what happens. If you eat yogurt and you get a breakout, then you know yogurt is your kryptonite. Some yogurts contain more sugar per serving than two donuts, so watch out.

Obviously if you're allergic to any of the ingredients in the smoothie list, you can substitute them for something else or leave that particular ingredient out completely. Don't eat something that'll hurt you just because it's on the list. Treat yourself well. This book is about health promotion and it would be a crying shame if you got sick because you ate something that you knew would be harmful to you.

So now you're probably thinking that you should be drinking nothing but smoothies for the rest of your life right? Wrong. The idea behind the smoothie is to give your body a starting point for healing. Smoothies are great, but don't be afraid to eat other foods also that are on the leafy green side. You can actually check out my website at www.epiphanyhealthcounseling.com/recipes for some great recipe ideas on top of what's in the recipe section of the book.

Root vegetables and mushrooms are also great for healing your acne and reducing inflammation. Root vegetables are things like carrots, onions, radishes, and other vegetables like potatoes. These root vegetables contain vitamins and minerals that help rebuild your body. Are you seeing the bigger picture yet? If you give your body the good stuff it needs, it'll treat you well and have a long operational lifespan.

Let's look at a car. Ferrari anyone? If you were to put kitchen oil in your engine, would your engine run? Not likely. You'd probably cause hundreds if not thousands of dollars' worth of damage. Cars are made to run on specific fuels to give them optimal performance. Bad fuel = bad performance. Your body is a lot like that car with one exception. Cars can't fix themselves and your body can. You are already pre-packaged with everything you need to repair yourself, but you have to put in the right fuel to make it work right. Your body only has one means of being able to get the right ingredients for rebuilding itself. It's through your food.

You are quite literally what you eat. Junk in, junk out. Whole foods in, you'll have a whole body. Good fuel = good performance. You can't go wrong with eating stuff that's truly from a tree or the ground assuming it's not poisonous. Poison Ivy is something you don't want to eat and does not apply to this example. Within reason though, if you can buy it at a supermarket, then you shouldn't have any problems. Now some people at this point may want to explore the topics of soil depletion, and nutrient deficiencies in plants caused by soil depletion.

To be honest, in my opinion, it's not something I would be too worried about right now if I were you. Some people use the excuse that they shouldn't eat vegetables and greens because the soil isn't good anymore to avoid eating foods they know they should be. I like using this example. Let's say you were to drop a nuclear bomb at a test site that was half as destructive as the biggest bomb you had in your arsenal. Does it matter that the nuclear devastation only went for two miles instead of four? No! Just because something isn't as potent as its full potential doesn't mean it's any less "destructive". Whole foods are like that example. Even though our current supply of vegetables is in some cases less potent than what they were decades ago, it doesn't mean they aren't effective today.

What is it about leafy greens and fruits that make them so good for you? First of all, they have a ton of nutrients, vitamins, and other chemicals that actually protect your cells from damage and rebuild anything that has already been damaged.

One of the means by which this is accomplished is through antioxidants. An antioxidant is the colored part of the fruit or vegetable. It's what gives produce its color. The ruby red of grapefruits, orange in carrots, red in apples, purple in grapes-you get the idea. Without these antioxidants, your body would begin to break down at an accelerated rate.

So what is an antioxidant exactly? Remember how we talked about the rust on the bumper on a car and how some people make snap judgments based on what they see? Rust starts on a bumper through a process called oxidation. Without getting too technical, oxidation happens when a material interacts with oxygen and loses an electron at the atomic level. In some cases it causes that substance to begin to break down. In other cases, it can actually be beneficial. In your body, things need to be in balance. Oxygen is great for a lot of things like...breathing. However, it can be problematic for you cells if it's all they are exposed to. Oxidation is what causes rust in metal, and causes the release of free radicals in your body. Free radicals can "radically" damage your cells lining and thus cause damage, minor or otherwise, to your organs.

Antioxidants stop that breakdown of your cells by giving your cells a protective lining in order to keep from losing their electrons and having the atoms gain a positive charge. That's why when you buy fresh fruit from the supermarket, it has a shelf life of a few days. The second you open that fruit the cells inside that fruit start to break down. The peel in the case of fruit acts as the "antioxidant". It keeps the fruit fresh on the tree and stops bacteria and other things from breaking through and prematurely breaking down the fruit.

There as an old joke that goes like this. Two atoms were in combat one day and one of them was hit. "I've lost an electron!" he yelled. The other responded, "Are you sure?" The electron that was hit adamantly replied, "I'm positive!" Okay so that was a really corny joke, but the idea is no less important.

Your body is incredibly efficient and functional. When it's in balance, it functions amazingly well, and is very robust and resilient. Your body handles a massive assault of toxins, germs, and viruses on a daily basis yet comes out on top almost every time. Dis-ease (disease) in any form be it acne, or something else, happens when the body is thrown out of balance. This is why oxygen isn't bad for you if it's kept in balance with antioxidants. The antioxidants stop you from "rusting".

Have you ever been to a mall or shopping center where you saw someone hawking some kind of skin care product that was derived from grapes? There may be some truth to what they're saying about it being good for your skin. Now I'm not advocating a grape cream to relieve your acne. The whole point of this book is to stress that pills, soaps, supplements, or creams are not necessary for acne reduction/elimination. However, if you feel you want to try any of these creams, then go for it. Please keep in mind though that many of these creams only have a "natural" label and not really natural ingredients. Remember too that creams are not necessary if you're doing the right things for your body. If you get antioxidant support from your food and you're drinking enough water, your skin will look as good or better than the cream can provide.

Back to the grape idea. The antioxidant in some grapes is called resveratrol. Recently, resveratrol has come under more scrutiny as some scientists have started saying that it's all hype and no science. These are the same people that have ignored other studies that show evidence for acne and diet being related. You'll often find resveratrol criticisms coming from these same people.

Resveratrol's potency comes from its ability to reduce inflammation[30]. Since acne is an inflamed area of your body, then resveratrol is probably a good thing to help reduce that inflammation. This is why some people swear by those grape creams. Really, if resveratrol comes from grapes, it's probably a good idea to get it directly from the source. Curiously enough, this might be why people that drink wine may have reduced risks for heart disease. Heart disease is also inflammation. Because science is barely starting to catch up with nutrition, the chemical reactions that happen with antioxidants in food are not well understood. There's a reason nature packed food the way it did on a tree or vine. If science tries to isolate these compounds from their

---

[30] http://articles.mercola.com/sites/articles/archive/2009/08/18/the-secrets-of-resveratrols-health-benefits.aspx

original packaging we don't know what can really happen good or bad.

The reactions between antioxidants, nutrients, and minerals in a fruit or vegetable are very interdependent. For example, there was hype over raspberry ketones at one point. The logic was that if ketones were this wonder substance in raspberries and you could only get so much by eating a few raspberries, then removing the ketones and putting them in a supplement form would have to be better for you. Right? Well, maybe but we don't really know. If one ketone supplement pill gives you the equivalent of 2 bowls of raspberries that doesn't mean it's better for you. There's a reason why nature won't let you typically eat so many raspberries in one sitting.

We are taught, that if something is good for you, then more of that thing must be better. That's like saying because your car's fuel tank can only hold 14 gallons, and your car gets you places you need to be, then you should put more gas in then that tank can handle.

See how this can be problematic? When your tank is full, it's full. When your body starts telling you, you shouldn't be eating anymore of something, you really need to stop. Nature knows how to package its food to support all life on this planet. We need to start trusting that process. Really, if you're not eating fruits and vegetable, it doesn't matter if they are at their full nutrient capacity. You are already severely deficient. Fun fact for you, your bones are like your body's bank account. Your bones, the place where your blood is created, are made up of vitamins and minerals. Whenever your body "spends" all your nutrients in your organs, it starts to make withdrawals from your bones. This is one of the reasons why people get achy bones. Their body is over drawing the account. This leads to issues with bone density and consequently issues with other parts of your body including your face. You need adequate nutrition. There is no other way to fully gain control of your acne without it.

Leafy greens and antioxidants aside, there are also some other essential foods that are necessary to restore your health in more places than just your face. These foods are so potent, they can even solve any emotional problem, stress problem, and contentment issue you may be having. So what do you do about the toxic emotional build up? I want to introduce you to another concept called *Primary Food* which includes Relationships, Career, Spirituality, and Physical Activity. Primary Food at its basic level, is the "real" food that nourishes your humanity. Vitamin-L is by far the most important vitamin in the world.

Without it, you can have some serious emotional and psychological consequences. A study was conducted with baby rhesus monkeys where they put a wire mockup of a rhesus monkey mother that gave milk to the monkey babies. Next to that, they put another mockup of a rhesus monkey mother with fur, but no food. The result? The baby rhesus monkeys spent most of their time in the arms of the furry mother over the wire mesh mother that provided food [31]. The furry mockup was a substitute for the lack of relationship the baby was experiencing. It sought Vitamin-L from an inanimate object that wasn't able to give it what it really needed. You may have guessed what Vitamin-L is by now. Love. Love nourishes you in so many profound ways. These "primary

---

[31] http://darkwing.uoregon.edu/~adoption/studies/HarlowMLE.htm

foods" nourish as much or more than the physical, secondary foods you are eating.

How does love help your acne? If you love yourself, then you are going to take steps to treat yourself well. You'll follow the steps in this book and get more than just your acne taken care of. You'll appreciate the person you are. If you're not loving yourself, that'll send stress through the roof and be shown all over your face. Acne or not, people will see the emotional toll of self-loathing and you not loving yourself.

If you enjoy your career, then you'll have far less stress at your job and more enjoyment of the tasks you have to do at that job. You can actually see an acne reduction coincide with feeling contentment in your career. Granted every job is going to have some measure of stress, regardless if you love it or not. But if you do love it and you get stressed there's something you can do to keep the love of your career alive.

You can exercise. That word has such negative connotations attached to it. What do you mean exercise? Whenever I've had some really big tasks ahead of me, a good run or even some jumping jacks really gets the blood pumping and makes me feel great. Getting the picture? Primary Foods reduce stress and self-loathing and give your body a rush of good hormones to bring it healing.

Spiritual practice is a sensitive topic for people, but regardless of what god you believe in, you as a person were made for spirituality. Everyone seeks out spirituality in one sense or another. We are always looking for someone, or something much higher than ourselves to answer to. For some people they answer to Jesus. For others they answer to science as their higher authority. Regardless, you will answer to something or someone greater than yourself.

Since that's the case it only makes sense that if you are discontented with your present spirituality, maybe it's time to either reconnect with that spirituality, or find something that you can truly, deeply connect with. I know this may sound a little too philosophical, but believe it or not, spirituality is always at play and has to be considered when we're looking at any health issue. It doesn't matter if it's acne, or stomach pain, all of these factors have to be taken into account when leading the body to wellness and healing

To recap, leafy greens, root vegetables, and plant based smoothies are essential to getting rid of your acne. Within the last 3 chapters we have talked about drinking water, cutting back on your dairy, how your health is individual to you, reducing/eliminating sugar, and eating other foods besides meat. We can't forget about the Primary Foods of Relationships, Career, Physical Activity, and Spirituality as playing a key role nourishing more than just our faces. Each of these things builds on the other. This is how we reset your body and get it to start bringing your acne under control.

If you haven't noticed by now. I've made no mention of any kind of product or supplement to help your acne. You really don't need any. If you follow the simple advice in this book, then you're body will do what it does best: it will keep you alive and vibrantly healthy and reduce if not eliminate your acne. What about life beyond acne? What happens after you take control?

Part Five:

Life Beyond Acne

14:
ACNE AND THE CHANGES OF LIFE

During your lifetime, if you've ever had a pimple, you are more than likely going to get another one. It doesn't matter if you're 12 years old or 52 years young, your body will get a pimple at some other point in time or another. How severe those pimples assert themselves though, doesn't have to be something that's a huge issue. Take for example a 50 year old woman that changes her facial cream, or switches her makeup. She'll more than likely get a pimple just like her 25 year old counterpart.

We've already gone into how makeup affects your face so I'm not trying to rehash that idea.

What about babies? Did you know even they can get acne? When a newborn first enters this world, their body undergoes a lot of changes the second they hit this atmosphere. They were tethered to mommy through the umbilical cord for so long, that their bodies start to do weird things hormonally. New born acne is actually quite common. Mom's hormones can do weird things to and now both of them can get acne. The good news is, if mom eats well, takes care of herself, nourishes her body with both Primary and Secondary foods, baby's acne will more than likely go away sooner than later. Once you get to the basics of how to control acne, it becomes easier and easier to get healthy.

The point of this whole book has been to teach you to take control of your acne and not have to abuse your body in the process.

Some of you in following these steps, will probably never have to deal with acne ever again. That is truly a very real possibility. Some of you, like me, may get the occasional pimple here and there if you do eat foods that cause flare ups. The overall mission each of us should be on, is to be healthy. If we concentrate first and foremost on our health, and not on a specific ailment like acne, then the rest of our body will be healthy and other issues will melt away like a fallen scoop of ice cream on side walk in 100 degree heat.

The more you love your body, the more it heals. It doesn't matter if you're 20 years old or 80 years old. Give yourself the life giving foods you need, and acne won't be able to eat your lunch like it's been doing most of your life. No pun intended.

My Acne Nightmare:

During my last pregnancy my skin looked great. After I delivered, maybe a week or two afterward both my newborn daughter and I started breaking out really bad. I acne on my chest and on my back. It seemed like nuts and greasy foods made my breakouts worse. Not having enough water did it also. It was kind of weird.

Jennifer's Story- 29 years old

15:
SO HOW LONG DOES THIS TAKE?

So how soon after following the advice in this book can you see a reduction/elimination of your acne? For some of you reading this, after cutting back on your dairy, sugar, and after you start drinking more water; you'll notice results in as little as two to seven days. If you keep up with the other pieces of advice in this book, like being aware of hormone laced foods, and crowding out any remaining health inhibiting foods with health promoting ones; you'll have full control of your acne in 30 days, and know how to keep it off without having to think about it.

For others, the time frame may be longer depending on how much toxicity is in your body. Some people can take two to six months to see their acne disappear off of their back for example, or it may even be two to three months for their face. My back and shoulder acne, took about three months to clear up once I followed this advice. Bio-Individuality will determine the time frame, but I stress that for the vast majority, relief will be very swift. Now I only get the occasional pimple and not the full breakout like I used to. Unfortunately I do have a lot of scarring on my face and back that I can't do much about right now. My face cleared up far faster than the rest of my body though. People noticed a huge difference more readily then if it was just on my back. It may be different for you though. Maybe the acne clears up on other parts of your body first and then your face.

Don't be discouraged if you don't see everything disappear overnight. It took a long time for your body to be damaged by environmental toxins and foods that are harmful. Really it took a lifetime if you think about it. It may take a little bit of time to let your body reset back where it needs to be. The good news is, you'll heal far faster than it took you to damage yourself. The body is amazingly and remarkably resilient. It can survive some of the most horrible things.

You may get faster clear ups with pills and products, but if you don't deal with the source of acne, you'll always be dependent on them. You'll be caught in the medicinal Cold War between stronger breakouts and stronger meds. It really isn't a good way to live. I've said this before, but why not take control of acne at its source? Why be dependent and have to spend money on acne for the rest of your life?

If you really want to do some reflection, how many things in your life have you survived-car accidents, deaths in the family, the emotional toll that sickness and disease can take on loved ones? Even the shame of having acne, is something that you've truly survived. For anyone that's been on the receiving end of being stared at because of how bad your face was, or anyone that was made fun of because of acne, I applaud you. You are truly a survivor. You survived that kind of pain with your mind intact, and your body going forward. Acne is not a sign of weakness, or lack of will power. Acne is something you have endured, and in spite of what it has done to you, you thrived.

This is what leads us to life truly beyond acne. I had a friend of mine that suffers from Lupus. She kept telling me how people treated her like a disease and not a person once they found out that she had it. From doctors to friends looking at her like she was some kind of leper, she rose up and took control of her disease, her confidence, and her sense of self. Her personal slogan was something like "I am not Lupus."

The power of that one statement is more than true. If you can get a hold of that kind of confidence and power, your body will respond by preparing itself to heal. Your mind will subconsciously make your body respond to the positive emotions and energy you are sending to it by taking away the hormones that cause stress and disease.

I want to tell you right now that you are not acne. You are more than acne. It can be a real pain to have people look at you and see nothing but a cratered swollen mass. Some people get acne so bad that it can obscure their vision.

Other people have acne so bad, it looks like burnt skin. This does not have to be you. Repeat this with me, "I am more than acne."

So what does life without acne look like? Imagine if you could look in the mirror and not be embarrassed to see the person staring back at you. Let me show you what life without acne looks like. When you can finally see your skin peak out from the shrinking mountains on your face it's an amazing feeling. Not having pimples pop on your back and bleed through your clothing, not having to rush to the bathroom when a pimple decides to burst before a board meeting, not having to deal with these things is really what's truly priceless.

If after following this book you don't get results, one of two things may be happening. First, your Bio-Individual body may not be allowing you to get relief, or there may be something wrong with you that goes deeper than food or stress. If that's the case, then it's not a failure on your part, and it's not that you didn't do things right. Rarely does someone fail to get relief; but, if it's the case that you don't, maybe it is an issue of genetics (extremely rare but possible), or it could even be the toxic environment you live in is not allowing your body to heal. Another side note on stress, if your life is highly stressful, it doesn't matter how much great medication, soap, or food you use, you will not see relief. That stress is actually a symptom of a greater problem or problems going on in your life. If that's the case I would suggest finding a trusted friend, loved one, or health professional that you can get help from to help you work through those issues. There's no shame in getting help, because really getting help is not a demonstration of your weakness. It's a demonstration of the powerful strength inside of you that says you are not afraid to tell someone you need help and you are strong enough to say something.

Most people are too weak to say anything to anyone about the issues they struggle with. Those are the people that never overcome anything. They're always stuck like a hamster in a wheel. Always running as fast as they can, but never really getting anywhere. Don't be that person. Speak up.

The second possibility is that you didn't try the concepts fully. You may be telling yourself that buying this book was a waste of your time.

If you go into something with blinders on and assume that it won't work for you, don't be surprised when it doesn't. Don't let ego, pride, or fear get in the way of truly experiencing relief. If you follow these simple concepts laid out in this book, and assuming your body will let you heal, you will see a reduction if not an elimination of your acne.

Imagine what it will feel like when you finally see a clear face staring back at you in the mirror. You've gotten control over something you were told that you had to live with for the rest of your life. It's a liberating feeling taking back your power from something so dark and bringing yourself back from the brink of despair. It's time to have a life beyond acne.

16:
THE POWER IS YOURS

This is what life beyond acne looks like-confidence, assurance, and a new found sense of self. Imagine what you would be able to do with that kind of confidence. One of the cool things of life beyond acne is that no matter how old you are, people won't be looking at you like you're a kid. Even up until I was 25, people still thought of me as a teenager. The acne did nothing to dissuade their assumptions. All people saw was a kid in big boy clothes trying to play house and be an adult.

As I have said before, it was really aggravating to try and sell life insurance and have your up-line tell you not to mess with or poke your face in front of other business people or your colleagues. He was an older gentleman, but it was still extremely embarrassing. Especially since I had such a hard time keeping it under control.

Now, people still think I look like a kid but it's not because I leak oil from my skin. It's actually because my skin has been rejuvenated and looks much younger and healthier than it ever did before. When I first began to reset my body internally, I went to Houston, Texas on a business trip. A friend of mine that I hadn't seen in a while came into his brother's house where I was staying and couldn't believe his eyes.

"Dude!" he said. "What did you do to your face?"

"What do you mean?" I replied.

"Your face man! You look ten years younger. I'm not kidding!"

It's true though. I had taken ten years off my face. It was a real eye opening experience. It created an interesting problem though. I already had trouble with people taking me seriously for my age. Now I really did look ten years younger. I started getting carded for buying glue for my piano tuning business. It has been both frustrating and empowering at the exact same time.

This entire journey started because I attended the world's largest nutrition school called the Institute for Integrative Nutrition. That's where I learned about Bio-Individuality, Primary Food and 100 different dietary theories and how to apply them in the human body. This was so helpful in understanding how with simple concepts, anyone, and I mean anyone can be taught to make themselves healthier and even heal their own bodies. They can be taught to listen to their body's innate voice and lift themselves out of disease.

Within the first 6 months of attending the school I had dropped 26 pounds in a healthy way, reversed my chronic fatigue, headaches, and lethargy. I had also managed to completely clear up my face. That's why my friend was so shocked. I need to stress that my back, arms, and chest took a little longer to clear up, but I can truly say that once they did, acne breakouts were a thing of the past.

Sure I do get the occasional pimple here and there, but as I mentioned earlier, it has more to do with eating foods that are sugary or high in hormones than genetics. If I enjoy the goodness of smoothies and leafy greens, then I have full control over my acne. If I hadn't done something about my health, acne would have been a constant companion beyond young adulthood and well into my 30's.

That's what this book has been about. Control-taking control of the uncontrollable. Mastering that which is said cannot be mastered. Life beyond acne is about being healthy in more ways than just your face. Just like acne is a symptom of the bigger problems happening in your body and life, a clear face is symptomatic of a life that is getting in order and health that is becoming more vibrant. Is that the life you want, or do you want a life of constant struggle without knowing what to do? You be the judge.

Part Six:

Additional Aids and Info

17:
RECIPES!

Orange Banana Blueberry Smoothie Blast

(Adapted from the Vitamix Cookbook)

Ingredients:

1 cup of water

1 orange, peeled and sectioned

1 frozen banana, previously peeled and chopped

½ to 1/3 cup frozen blueberries

Instructions:

Combine all of the ingredients in a blender and blend for 30 to 45 seconds or until a smoothie like consistency is achieved.

Green Smoothie

(Adapted from the Vitamix Cookbook)

Ingredients:

Around 1/2 cup of coconut water or regular water (your choice)

1/2 cup of pineapple juice

1/2 of a pear or apple

1/2 cup of spinach leaves (not the frozen kind)

1 broccoli floret

1/2 an avocado

1-2 cups of green grapes.

1 cup of ice

Tools:

Cutting Board

Knife

Blender

To Make The Smoothie:

Chop all of the grapes, broccoli floret, pear/apple into small pieces.

Pour the water and juice into the blender.

Cut the avocado in half and put that half in the blender making sure to leave out the peel.

Pour the grapes, broccoli, and pear/apple into the blender.

Add the ice and start the blender on the ice crushing setting for about 40 seconds or until a smooth consistency is achieved.

Enjoy!

Portobello Mushroom Steaks

(Inspired by the Institute for Integrative Nutrition)

Ingredients:

4 large portobello mushrooms

2 ½ teaspoons oregano

2 ½ tablespoons balsamic vinegar

2 tablespoons olive oil

¼ teaspoon garlic powder

Salt and pepper to taste

Instructions:

Preheat oven to 350 degrees

Wash full mushrooms with stems and then remove the stems

Mix the olive oil, oregano, garlic powder, and balsamic vinegar in a dish.

Place mushrooms and stems in an edged backing dish and pour oil mixture over mushrooms, making sure to cover them as much as possible.

Bake for 25-30 minutes and serve

Enjoy!

Steve's Vegetable Medley

(My Original Recipe)

Ingredients:

2 celery stocks, chopped

¼ to ½ cup mushrooms

½ red onion, chopped

2 carrots, chopped

3 garlic cloves, minced

6 broccoli florets, chopped

Bragg's Liquid Aminos

Instructions:

Combine garlic, onion, 4-5 squirts of liquid aminos, and mushrooms into a pan over medium heat.

Sautee mixture until mushrooms and onions just start to get soft

Add remaining carrots, celery and broccoli and continue cooking over medium heat for another 5-7 minutes.

Serve and enjoy!

Stephen's Tomato Vegetable Soup:

(My Original Recipe)

Ingredients:

1 Pacific™ Tomato Soup (or similiar product)

3-5 Broccoli florets chopped

8 oz of Mushrooms chopped

1/3 Red Onion chopped

2 garlic cloves chopped

1/8 cup cilantro stemmed

1-2 carrots sliced

2 Green onion stalks, chopped (optional)

3 dashes of Turmeric

3 dashes of Curry

Black Pepper and Salt to taste

Instructions:

1. Begin to heat Soup over medium heat

2. Sauté Mushrooms, garlic cloves, and Onions until mushrooms begin to release their juices. Add Broccoli and carrots and continue for about 3-5 minutes.

3. Add vegetable mixture to soup, stir, and turn up heat to med-high.

4. Add cilantro, turmeric, curry, pepper, and salt. Stir and add additional spices to taste

5. When Soup begins to slightly boil serve immediately.

Cabbage and Peach Carrot Smoothie

(Adapted from the Vitamix Cookbook)

Ingredients:

1/3 cup water

¾ cup sliced green cabbage

1 to 1-1/4 cup green grapes

1 halved and pitted peach

1 chopped carrot

1/3 cup ice

Instructions:

Slice the cabbage

Halve and pit the peach

Chop the carrot

Place all ingredients into a blender and blend together on high for 30 to 45 seconds, or until a smoothie like consistency is achieved.

18:
REFERENCES AND RESOURCES

Bershad SV, "Diet and acne—slim evidence, again, J Am Acad Dermatol (2005);53(6): p. 1102; author reply p. 1103

http://www.aad.org/stories-and-news/news-releases/growing-evidence-suggests-possible-link-between-diet-and-acne

http://www.medscape.com/viewarticle/722953_3

http://johnsern.articlealley.com/the-history-of-acne-223237.html

http://www.aqhealth.com/skin-care/acne-treatment/history-of-acne-egyptian-roman-greek-perspective-2300.html

http://www.cdc.gov/getsmart/antibiotic-use/antibiotic-resistance-faqs.html#how-bacteria-resist

http://www.ncbi.nlm.nih.gov/pubmed/7784640

http://www.webmd.com/drugs/2/drug-6661/accutane-oral/details#side-effects

http://columbia.legalexaminer.com/fda-prescription-drugs/controversy-ridden-accutane-pulled-from-pharmacy-shelves/

http://www.webmd.com/drugs/2/drug-5919-73/tetracycline-oral/tetracycline-oral/details#side-effects

http://www.webmd.com/drugs/2/drug-20405/benzaclin-top/details#side-effects

http://www.webmd.com/drugs/2/drug-95358-5115/yaz-28-oral/ethinylestradiol-drospirenone-oral/details#side-effects

http://umm.edu/health/medical/altmed/supplement/vitamin-b12-cobalamin

http://www.staffanlindeberg.com/TheKitavaStudy.html

http://archderm.jamanetwork.com/article.aspx?articleid=479093

http://healthland.time.com/2011/05/16/could-a-spoonful-of-sugar-help-the-medicine-work/

http://ajcn.nutrition.org/content/94/2/479.long

http://www.ncbi.nlm.nih.gov/pubmed/15692464

http://articles.mercola.com/sites/articles/archive/2008/01/02/dairy-industry-self-destructs.aspx

http://www.organicconsumers.org/articles/article_5543.cfm

http://www.ncbi.nlm.nih.gov/pmc/articles/PMC1257574/

http://www.scientificamerican.com/article/where-does-blue-food-dye/

http://www.fda.gov/Cosmetics/Labeling/IngredientNames/ucm109084.htm

http://science.howstuffworks.com/environmental/energy/oil-refining2.htm

http://ec.europa.eu/consumers/cosmetics/cosing/index.cfm?fuseaction=search.results&annex_v2=II&search

http://www.fda.gov/iceci/inspections/inspectionguides/ucm074952.htm

http://www.ncbi.nlm.nih.gov/pubmed/16922622

http://www.fda.gov/iceci/inspections/inspectionguides/ucm074952.htm

http://www.nbcnews.com/id/16614865/ns/us_news-life/t/woman-dies-after-water-drinking-contest/

http://articles.mercola.com/sites/articles/archive/2009/08/18/the-secrets-of-resveratrols-health-benefits.aspx

http://darkwing.uoregon.edu/~adoption/studies/HarlowMLE.htm

ABOUT THE AUTHOR

Stephen Rodriguez is a speaker, author, holistic health coach, musical artist, and pastor that specializes in teaching disease and premature death prevention while getting people motivated to love themselves and live up to their full potential in every area of their spirit, soul, and body. Having suffered with the stigma and shame of acne for many years, *Clear You: Acne Healing Solution* is written to show you, the reader, how to get control of your acne, and establish a foundation for true and lasting health beyond clear skin. You are worthy to thrive!

CPSIA information can be obtained at www.ICGtesting.com
Printed in the USA
LVOW04s2317250115

424266LV00044B/1566/P